Green Smoothie Bliss™

The __Ultimate Guide__ To Make Smart Green Smoothies For Whole-Body Healing

Rhonda E. Alexander, M.S., M.A.
Certified Fitness Trainer (CFT)
Specialist in Fitness Nutrition (SFN)

Part of the *Live Younger, Longer and Prettier!*™ series

ISSA
The World Leader In
ISSA
International Sports Sciences Association
Fitness Certification
Since 1988
CERTIFIED

ISBN: 978-1-63263-391-0

Published by Quintessential Publishing Company, Inc., Chicago, IL

Printed in the United States of America.

Quintessential Publishing Company, Inc.
2014

First Edition

Dedication

Thank you God for all that you've given me and all that you've protected me from. Because of the many challenges along the way to completing this project, I had no choice except to sit down and get this playbook done on my own. Now I see this is how it was supposed be all along. Everyone has his/her own journey, and I'm grateful for mine.

This book is dedicated to my mom, who is a fighter, an overcomer and a soon-to-be cancer survivor–I just know it. In the midst of everything we have endured, over the last few years especially, you've been my rock. I pray God grants me the opportunity to repay you just a smidgeon of what you've given to me for my entire life. Any hair-brained scheme I came up with, you've been there for me, supporting me in any way you could, until I ultimately found the love of my professional life: writing. Whether it is ghostwriting, one of my fictional tales of intrigue (wink), or penning articles about health and wellness and now this full-length recipe guide – you've been the best cheerleader anyone could wish for. You may have given me the side eye every time I produced one of my green smoothie "concoctions" for you to try, but you kept encouraging me to keep going and refine my recipes with constructive criticism, which was invaluable. Having just one person believe that I could do whatever I set my mind to doing has made all the difference. Your support gave me the confidence to believe in myself. I have no idea where I would be without my God and without you.

I love you mommy,

Rhonda

Disclaimer

The term "green" is used to express ingredients that are highly nutritious and being the closest form to nature, or "of the earth" versus other recipes consumer may have tried that are filled with artificial ingredients. Some of these recipes can be highly caloric. The smoothies are meant to replace meals, not accompany them. If consumed in addition to regular meals, count on adding weight to your frame. Many of the author's clients use these recipes on a short-term basis to jumpstart their fat and weight loss as well as discipline their eating habits.

***Author's advice:** pay close attention to the **nutritional data** supplied with these recipes for meal planning purposes and **nutritional needs**. As always, the advice in this manual is not intended to treat or diagnose any condition or disorder.*

While the author's attempt is to be as accurate as possible, it should not be relied upon as being comprehensive.

Use of the information contained in this book does not constitute a doctor-patient relationship.

The information presented in this booklet is not intended to diagnose, treat or cure disease.

Please discuss this information with your own physician or healthcare provider to determine what is right for you. The information presented here is intended for general knowledge only and should not be used as a substitute for medical advice or treatment.

Author cannot and does not give medical advice. The information contained in this book is presented in summary form only and is intended to provide broad consumer understanding and knowledge as well as provide the consumer with a base of knowledge to empower them to be an advocate and CEO of their own health versus simply accepting what practitioners dispense as the only path for wellness.

This information should not be considered complete and should not be used in place of a visit, call, consultation, or advice of health care provider. Author does not recommend the self-management of health problems.

Information obtained through Live Younger, Longer and Prettier sites (self-help series, blog, e-book, book and all forms of social media) are not exhaustive and do not cover all diseases, ailments, physical conditions, or treatments.

Should you have any health care questions, call or see your physician or other health care provider promptly. Never disregard medical advice or delay in seeking it because of something shared within the entities of Green Smoothie Bliss or the Live Younger, Longer and Prettier series of self-help books. While the author's goal is to empower you to make better decisions for your health, the author is still an advocate of working with your healthcare provider to arrive at the best course of treatment for your medical condition.

This book details the author's personal experiences with and opinions about making low carb, nutritious green smoothies. The author is not a healthcare provider.

The author and publisher are providing this book and its contents on an "as is" basis and make no representations or warranties of any kind with respect to this book or its contents. The author and publisher disclaim all such representations and warranties, including for example warranties of merchantability and healthcare for a particular purpose.

The statements made about products and services have not been evaluated by the U.S. Food and Drug Administration. They are not intended to diagnose, treat, cure, or prevent any condition or disease.

Please consult with your own physician or healthcare specialist regarding the suggestions and recommendations made in this book.

Except as specifically stated in this book, neither the author or publisher, nor any authors, contributors, or other representatives will be liable for damages arising out of or in connection with the use of this book. This is a comprehensive limitation of liability that applies to all damages of any kind, including (without limitation) compensatory; direct, indirect or consequential damages; loss of data, income or profit; loss of or damage to property and claims of third parties.

You understand that this book is not intended as a substitute for consultation with a licensed healthcare practitioner, such as your physician. Before you begin any healthcare program, or change your lifestyle in any way, you will consult your physician or other licensed healthcare practitioner to ensure that you are in good health and that the examples contained in this book will not harm you.

This book provides content related to topics physical and/or mental health issues. As such, use of this book implies your acceptance of this disclaimer.

Contents

Preface

Hello Green Smoothie lovers!

Are you ready to find your bliss? Your green smoothie bliss, that is …

Thank you so much for allowing me to be a part of your wellness journey. Thank you for trusting me to share information I've learned along the way, through research, studying, experimentation and interviews, but mostly trial and error, as I discovered my own green smoothie bliss.

There's no shortage of information about making smoothies on the World Wide Web, but I noticed, a lot of the recipes don't disclose the carb content. The reason is most likely because the carb content is through the roof, in many cases. Some of the recipes I found during my research had over 100 carbs in one recipe, with no serving suggestions or precautions! That many carbs might send a diabetic to the hospital, if consumed all at once.

This guide started out with me looking for ways to enjoy fruity drinks, which have always been my weakness, in a healthier way. As a child, I loved a particular strawberry flavored milk drink, but as an adult, I found out the powder was nothing but sugar. When I checked the label, I found the delicious strawberry drink was a whopping 150 calories, in an 8-ounce serving (and let's be real, who drinks only 8-ounces of something delicious at one time?), 15 grams of carbs and zero nutrients.

By the time I reached my mid-thirties, my doctor had begun to talk to me about starting diabetic medication since my blood sugar level was high every time I went for a visit and my weight was getting out of control. My 5'3" frame was carrying over 180lbs of weight and all the exercising in the world was not making a lasting dent. When I refused the diabetic meds, she gave me six months to get my weight under better control, which she thought would stabilize my blood sugar. Giving up those sugary drinks that I loved was the hardest habit to break. Because the cravings for my fruity drinks didn't go away, I turned to the Internet to find answers and began to learn about using fruits and vegetables to make *healthy* fruit drinks. That's when my journey to *Green Smoothie Bliss* began.

I started making green smoothies to get control of my health, but along the way, it's become much more. Not only have I created recipes that allow me to enjoy fruity drinks in a healthier way, the low-carb options actually taste better than the processed, sugary drinks I'd grown addicted to over the years.

A big bonus was that I lost 38 lbs with this one tweak in my lifestyle: cutting out sugary, store-bought drinks. Then I began to discover just how influential vegetables, fruits, herbs and spices could be to improving other areas of my health. I began experimenting even more with different recipes that targeted complaints I heard from friends, family members and even social media contacts. The pages of *Green Smoothie Bliss* soon filled up with recipes containing foods that were known to target complaints, such as low energy, inflammation, muscle soreness, insomnia, low sex-drive, bad skin, bloating and so much more.

That's why it's taken over 16 months to bring this book from conception to publication. I couldn't stop myself!

I decided to pursue my certification in personal training and fitness nutrition in an effort to construct healthful recipes using whole foods that were known to target health conditions that plagued so many people I knew and loved. As I learned more, I couldn't stop experimenting with recipes and I delighted in my findings that green smoothies can do so much more than help you lose water weight.

Yes, I said it. ***Water Weight****.*

There are a lot of books out there claiming to detox you with green smoothies, promising you'll lose X amount of pounds in X amount of days, but come on folks. You're intelligent. You already know that if you stop eating solid foods for any amount of time, you will lose weight. You also know, and have maybe even experienced this for yourself, that the minute you stop the "smoothie diet/detox/flush" and begin reintroducing solid foods to your system, that weight is coming right back.

So I want to make it clear that this guide does NOT claim to help you lose weight by doing ALL green smoothies, ALL the time. No one can do that. I will claim that when you treat your body right by putting good food, with good nutrients, in it, your body will be good to you. The **best detox** is feeding your body well. That will ultimately help all the systems that are already in place (liver, kidneys, lymph nodes) for that purpose (to detox) do their job even better.

However, there is a right time to consume your smoothie to reduce the likelihood of it converting to stored calories the moment you consume it. Yep, there is a "guilt-free" time of the day to consume your green smoothies. Personal trainers may get upset with me for "spilling the tea," but oh well! There are still many more health secrets kept in the fitness community, so this is one they can just release because I'm giving it to you.

I also offer that watching the amount of carbs you put in your green smoothie will help you watch your weight. Since many people have an aversion to liquid vegetables -- at least I did when I first began making smoothies -- a gradual transition to a green smoothie that is low-carb, yet still very tasty will help you make smart, green smoothies too. The tips and short cuts I provide for you will make your transition very easy.

Part I
Introduction

Whether you want to release the "winter sludge," or you want to transition to a healthier lifestyle, adding green smoothies to your regimen can improve your life if you're willing to consider a few simple guidelines to help you make the most of your green smoothies.

1. There's a right time to consume green smoothies that can maximize calorie usage
2. Green smoothies made with whole foods, herbs and spices are best for your health
3. Don't be afraid to experiment and be open to new flavor combinations
4. Share high-carb recipes (more than 50 carbs) to continue to enjoy higher carb, green smoothies while you transition to low-carb, green smoothies

I'm sure you know someone who decided to incorporate green smoothies into their lifestyle thinking they would lose weight only to later have them report that not only have they not lost weight, they've actually GAINED WEIGHT!

How disappointing is that?

Many people think just because they are putting vegetables and fruits into their smoothies, it must be healthy. This must be the ticket to weight loss, and green smoothies are the answer they've been looking for. However, it's very important to realize that there is a SCIENCE to making a nutritious smoothie that is delicious, simple and good for your health.

Smoothie maker beware – the higher the calories in the ingredients, the higher your caloric intake will be and if your mission is to release extra weight, you must be careful of every ingredient you add to these recipes.

As one of my doctors put it, "Fruit is nature's candy and you have to be just as careful about the amount of fruit you consume as you do processed sugars like taffy and potato chips."

How is Green Smoothie Bliss different?

While there are a lot of low-cost and free books out there with tons of recipes in them, I want to tell you exactly what makes this one ***different***.

I have compiled these recipes so those who have little to no experience making healthy, green smoothies can begin to enjoy them without the trial and error you would endure trying to make recipes with foods you aren't sure about mixing together.

I've also arranged them in order – high, medium and low-carb – for those with carb sensitivities to gradually and naturally adjust to the reduction of carbs in green smoothies and still enjoy them. The recipes here provide a healthy alternative to a sit down meal or snack that tastes great and satiates your appetite for two to four hours.

Make no mistake – you're not supposed to use green smoothies as your only food source, by any means. The most I would encourage is to use green smoothies as two or three of the 10 servings of fruits and vegetables you should consume every day.

GSB starts out with recipes that have more ingredients in them, which masks the taste of the vegetables and makes them easier to tolerate for those who may initially find veggies such as, Swiss chard, kale and even spinach hard to swallow in liquid form.

Carb Requirements for Women and Men

Take note of the carb content and the calorie content – from the first recipe through the last – you will note that the calorie and carb content contains a high enough count to be considered a snack or a meal. If your goal is to lose weight, don't eat again until you're due for your next **meal** after you consume a smoothie that contains at least 45 carbs for women; for men, 60 carbs is allowed.

Exceptions to the Rule

There's one group of people who may require more than the normal amount of carbs per meal than the rest of us: Athletes. Especially right after a competition or a training session.

Athletes must immediately replace lost carbohydrates because they build glycogen (stored carbs), which is the storage fuel for muscles. After working out, muscles are able to store more glycogen than before working out. That storage of glycogen keeps athletes from becoming fatigued. Especially since they may be on diets that are lower in carbs as they prepare for competition and in many cases, much lower than they should actually be consuming.

To benefit from this principle, even if you aren't an athlete, consuming a higher carb smoothie, balanced with protein within 90-minutes of a rigorous workout allows your body to use up the extra carbs right away to replenish carbs during that time. This is only recommended if you're pushing your workout to the max. You'll also need to replenish 24-ounces of water per pound of weight lost during a workout as immediate "weight" lost during a workout is not fat, but fluid.

Best time to consume smoothies and enjoy "guilt-free" carbs

Keeping in mind, the "exceptions to the rule" principle above, the best time to enjoy a smoothie with a higher carb content is right after a hard workout. Prepare your ingredients before your workout, so you won't lose time when you're finished. Once you have finished your workout, pop your ingredients in the blender and enjoy. You'll notice I didn't suggest blending your ingredients and refrigerating the smoothie beforehand.

Pre-blending your smoothie is a personal choice. I don't recommend it because, once the cell walls of the vegetables have been broken, the enzymes immediately begin to "die." If the enzymes are dying for an hour or more, by the time you return to consume your smoothie, you've lost the opportunity to optimize the benefits of the nutrients. There's no hard and fast scientific evidence as to how much of the enzymes are still viable, but I prefer not to guess. I know that if I blend just before I drink, the enzymes are at their peak of viability. This is why I recommend waiting to blend until you're actually ready to drink. There are differing schools of opinion on this, but mine is to blend just before consumption.

Foundational Green Smoothie Weight Loss Jumpstart Formula

Yes, I know, a couple of sections ago, I shared my disdain for the popular green smoothie diets that claim to help you shed pounds. It's true; the weight loss is normally temporary; and the weight lost is normally water weight that comes back as soon as you return to your regular diet. However, I do believe there is merit to what I refer to as a "foundational green smoothie weight loss jumpstart formula."

Sounds unnecessarily complicated, I know, but hear me out. I offer, that if you use this formula, you actually *can* have lasting weight loss.

It involves a lifestyle change after the jumpstart, but that's really the point of it all, isn't it? You want to make a change *for the better, for good,* not just a temporary 'quick fix' right?

Here's the formula:

For no more than five days at a time, exchange two of your five daily meals for low-carb smoothies. Use any of the recipes in the low-carb section you like; however, if the recipes have 45g-60g (medium-carb) of carbohydrates, limit consumption to half of the recipe you're making at a time. Because I recommend drinking your smoothie right after blending for the best chance of absorbing the living nutrients, plan to share a green smoothie that exceeds the recommended number of carbohydrates in a given recipe (or just make half the recipe). For those recipes that contain 25g-35g of carbs or lower, you may consume the entire volume for your meal. Carb counts between 36g-44g should be excluded during the 'jumpstart' period even though they may be tempting. The same recommendation applies for any recipe in the high-carb section unless you're splitting it in half as I recommended for the medium-carb (45g-60g) recipes above.

Also, incorporate the formula I shared earlier about the best time to consume your highest carb meal of the day, which is within 90-minutes of your toughest workout that day. At that point, you may burn up the majority of the calories you consume due to glycogen restoration and the 'afterburn' effect. Your two snacks, which are part of your five daily meals, should contain no more than 15g of carbs. I followed this formula and lost 12lbs. over a 10-day period, but of course, results may vary for everyone. In addition, I also converted my meals to contain no animal protein during this time as well. It was a challenge, to say the least; but because I was ready to transition to a diet that excluded meat, I was excited to see just how ready I was. This worked for me, but the goal is to find out where your "bliss" lies.

What is the most flavorful fruit to add to green smoothies?

I will preface this by agreeing, yes, it is a matter of opinion. Depending on your taste buds, certain fruits may taste more flavorful than others. Since I've been actively working on these green smoothie recipes for 16-months, I'm pretty confident about my findings in this regard.

I have to say, it was difficult for me to admit this fruit was the most flavorful of them all because I actually didn't care for the taste of them for most of my life. Nope it's not bananas. I didn't care for the taste of that fruit either and I still can't eat a banana without blending it in my smoothie. It's not apples either, as much as I hate to admit this since apples are my all-time favorite fruit.

The fruit I've found to add the most flavor to green smoothies is actually pears!

It stands to reason pears would pack a punch of flavor since they contain 26 carbs in one small pear. As I claimed earlier, I've been experimenting with these recipes for 16-months and pears are the only fruit I've found that I can use alone with any vegetable I choose and not need to add another fruit, such as pineapple or banana the way I ordinarily would. Using other fruits in my recipes serves to add variety, otherwise this book would be much shorter; you could simply use a pear, a green vegetable and call it a day!

A brief explanation of juicing versus smoothies

We think we're doing the right thing by juicing vegetables, but vegetables convert to carbohydrates when they are juiced (which is totally different from a smoothie, and is worth the mention since a lot of people juice and incorporate the juices into their smoothies) as juicers separate the fiber from the natural sugars in these awesome, life-enhancing foods.

The sugar is readily available, which makes it act like a simple sugar. It goes directly to your bloodstream instead of having to go through the systems in your body to get broken down and eventually make it to your bloodstream. Juices can make it to your bloodstream within 15 minutes versus an hour or longer for solid foods and other foods with fiber in them. If your body isn't ready to use the sugar right away, it gets stored.

Depending on your activity level, the sugar will be stored and used as it should be used. However, if you're not active, the sugar (as well as proteins, if consumed in excess) will be stored in the body where they will convert to fat if it isn't utilized properly (within an hour of consumption).

You need to increase the vegetables in your smoothies because you want to get as close to a true, green smoothie as you can in order to enjoy the benefits that come with consuming more vegetables; such as balanced pH levels, which are essential for optimal health.

Some people can tolerate all vegetable smoothies, some people can't; but never fear, if you find you need fruit in your smoothie, you'll still enjoy the benefits of consuming more vegetables in your diet. In fact, you'll find that if you combine green smoothies with an active lifestyle, and consume them at the right time, you can enjoy green smoothies with a modest amount of fruit in them and not have to pay the consequences (i.e. gaining weight and sustained high blood sugar levels, which put you at risk for Type 2 diabetes).

Liquid options

Use any liquid that you like. Let's face it. We all have certain flavors that we prefer, however, be aware that choosing a different liquid means you will have to pay a higher price: more calories. Listed below each recipe, you will find the calorie content of the various liquids you may decide to use in your green smoothie.

Eight ounces	Calories
Unsweetened Almond Milk	60
Vanilla almond milk	90
Coconut Water	45
Skim milk	80
Soymilk	100
Hemp milk	100
1% milk	110
2 % milk	130
Rice milk	120
Vanilla rice milk	130
Oat milk	130
Whole milk	150
Coconut Milk	120

Tips and short cuts to help you prepare your smoothies with ease:

- Ginger - Peel and cut in chunks and store in a bag in the freezer. Use a cheese grater to add ginger to smoothies. It breaks the tough, fibrous strands and makes the nutrient available to the cells of the body
- Bananas - Peel, store in individual snack bags and freeze - helps retain more flavor without watering down smoothies with ice cubes
- Greens - Blanche, let cool, store in individual portions in snack bags and freeze
- Veggie Water - Save from blanched greens to use as liquid for smoothies, but use within 1 day
- Fresh Pineapples -Turn upside down until you're ready to cut them. Storing the pineapples upside down helps the sweet juices distribute throughout the pineapple; that way, all of the pineapple is sweet instead of just the bottom, which is where the juices naturally flow
- Save your berries from the trash! If you can't eat them before they start to spoil, rinse them with 1 part ACV (apple cider vinegar) and 2 parts water. The ACV kills the bacteria that live on the berries and cause them to spoil so quickly. Fill ice trays with water and pop a berry or two per cube and freeze. Store your cubes in snack bags for convenience

Elements of a smart, green smoothie

All green smoothies that have a goal of improving your health contain four to five elements. Listed below is a chart to simplify the categories:

Elements of a Smart Green Smoothie

	Preferred	**Secondary**	
Vegetables	**Greens** (spinach, kale, Swiss chard, arugula, romaine lettuce, etc.)	**More Greens** (celery, turnip greens, beet greens, mustard, collards, etc.)	
Carbohydrates	**Fruits** (pineapple, pear, banana, etc.)	**Sweeteners** (honey, agave, molasses, etc.)	
Protein	**Plant-based Veg/Nuts/Nut Butters** (peanut butter, almond butter, sunflower seed butter, etc.)	**Powder** (flavored/unflavored protein powder, etc.)	
Fats	**Nuts, Seeds, Avocado** (sunflower seeds, almonds, pistachio, etc.)	**Oils** (coconut oil, avocado oil, sunflower oil, etc.)	
Liquid	**Water/herbal tea** (unsweetened)	**Nut Milk** (almond, coconut)	**Rice/Soy Milk**

Nutrient notes

Fat content is only listed in recipes where the fat grams are above 4g in the recipe.

Any recipe that doesn't list a specific liquid to add, use 6-8 ounces of filtered or alkaline water to maintain the caloric and carbohydrate content listed in the recipe.

All recipes contain some vitamin C, which is a natural antioxidant; therefore, each recipe included in this guide is considered an antioxidant-rich recipe.

Due to the grapefruit content in the citrus juice mix*, please double check for drug interaction if you are on cholesterol or blood pressure lowering medication.

***Citrus Juice Mix – Use a citrus juicer to extract the juice from:**

Juice of 1 lemon
Juice of 2 limes
1 medium-sized, pink grapefruit
1 medium-sized orange
One 1-inch piece of raw ginger (peel and freeze first and use cheese grater to grate into juice mix)

Mix juices together and refrigerate, but use within three days

Part II
High-Carb Smoothie Recipes

It's true carbohydrates are the body's main source of energy. Carbohydrates feed the muscles of the body, which helps keep you energized and functioning, from running errands to working out, to picking up the kids to going up a flight of stairs. The more rigorous the activity you perform, the more you need to replenish the body with the appropriate balance of carbs and protein to ensure there is muscle growth as well as replenishment of energy stores.

The following recipes for high-carb smoothies contain 60g of carbs and above. The **only** group of people who should even consider consuming an entire recipe in one serving are those who compete in endurance sports for more than 90 minutes at a time. At best, the high-carb smoothies contained in this section should be split in half and consumed at two different meal times. Sharing the other half is another great option.

Stoked Start Strudel

(Blood pressure/sugar regulator, digestion, gas relief, heart health)

½-cup oats
8 ounces of almond milk
1 tsp. vanilla extract
1 frozen banana
1 tsp. peanut butter
¼ tsp. cinnamon
¼ tsp. nutmeg

Calorie and Nutrition Count

Calories - 694
Carbs - 95g
Protein - 24g
Fat - 25g
Fiber - 15g
Vitamin A - 12mg
Vitamin C - 17mg

Ingredient Spotlight

Oats

There are three different types of oats: steel cut, rolled and instant. The biggest difference between them lies in the amount of processing that takes place. The more the oats are processed, the less fiber content they have and content truly is king in this instance. A cup of steel cut oats at the beginning of your day can keep you full, focused and fat-free for hours!

According to the Whole Grains Council, the fiber in oats keeps you satiated as well as keeps your blood pressure and bad cholesterol in check. Diabetics would do well to make oats a regular part of their diet as oats help to stabilize blood sugar levels.

Man Yana Nirvana

(Energy boost, digestion)

1-cup of spinach
1-cup mango
3 prunes
1 banana
4 ounces fresh squeezed orange juice
2 ounces lemon juice
4 ounces alkaline water

Calorie and Nutrition Count

Calories - 350
Carbs - 90g
Protein - 5g
Fiber - 12g
Vitamin A - 89mg
Vitamin C - 309mg

Ingredient Spotlight

Prunes

I've always thought of prunes as a giant raisin, but there's a lot more to them than that. They're actually dried plums, but in addition to being so much juicier than raisins, they also have a well-deserved reputation for improving regularity, but that's not all! After resolving digestive issues, the B vitamins put you in a great mood and you'll also enjoy an increase in energy levels. Who doesn't need a natural energy boost by the time 2 p.m. rolls around? They are high on the carb side at 26 grams per serving (about 5), but if you put them in the freezer to chill on a hot, summer day, you can enjoy them solo and still qualify as a low-carb treat.

Elvis N Da Building

(Energy, digestion)

2 tbsp. peanut butter
8 ounces vanilla almond milk
1 tsp. honey or agave nectar
1 tbsp. ground walnuts mixture
1 frozen banana

Calories and Nutrition

Calories - 520
Carbs - 68g
Protein - 14g
Fat - 25g
Fiber - 7g
Vitamin A - 21mg
Vitamin C - 15mg

Ingredient Spotlight

Almonds

I am allergic to certain varieties of seafood, but I feel awful for those who are allergic to nuts! There are so many vital benefits to adding all different types of nuts to your health regimen; I couldn't imagine my life without them.

Almonds happen to be my favorite nut of them all. Initially, it was because they tasted so delicious. As a child, mom would treat me to cinnamon covered almonds from a kiosk in the mall. We always seemed to get a fresh batch that was still warm (maybe that was a heating lamp, I don't know!) and this made them taste even better, somehow. Afterwards, we'd be energized and reinvigorated for the next leg of our day of shopping or errands. By the time we arrived home, we'd gotten in our exercise and stimulated our digestive system, which made for an incredibly satisfying "smooth move," yet another benefit of eating almonds.

Now I realize that spicy treat came with health benefits, such as increased brainpower and a boost of energy. Almonds contain elements that actually stimulate your brain and help you focus in addition to providing protection against certain diseases, such as Alzheimer's.

Almonds also help lower bad cholesterol and raise the good kind as well as protecting you from heart attacks due to the magnesium content. They are like one-stop shopping for better health from head-to-toe.

From your head to your heart and all the way down to your bones, the multiple benefits of almonds can't be denied. Eating them on a regular basis brings to mind those amazing cuffs worn by Wonder Woman. When Linda Carter spun around and magically changed from the demure military intelligence officer or nurse, depending on which incarnation of the story you're familiar with, those cuffs became her defense against bullets and anything bad coming her way. That's how I feel when I think of all the benefits associated with consuming almonds on a regular basis.

Bonus tips/recipes: I've even replaced traditional cow's milk with almond milk and created my own recipe for use in my smoothies and nondairy ice cream as well as a healthy drink to enjoy.

Homemade almond milk with no preservatives: Use 2 cups of almonds, ½ cup peanuts, 3 cups of alkaline water and a dash of kosher salt to the blender. Mix until you reach a smooth consistency, refrigerate and enjoy cold. If you'd like your milk thinner, add more water. If you want to have it right away, feel free to add a few ice cubes to make it even more refreshing.

Homemade nondairy ice cream with no preservatives: Use above recipe, add less water (2 cups, or even less, depending on how many other ingredients you add) and a frozen banana to the blender. Freeze for a nondairy, delicious ice cream. Add extracts and other flavorings, such as apricot extract, vanilla extract, almond extract or any flavoring that suits your fancy. Feel free to incorporate your favorite fruits, such as sliced, frozen strawberries, peaches, mango, lychee, or whatever fruit you'd like, it's up to your taste buds!

Switch it up and add 2 cups of shredded coconut instead of almonds or mix half and half (half almonds, half coconut) to experiment and find the perfect flavor for you!

Peach Party Fantasy

(Folic acid, eyesight protectant, wound healer)

1-cup pineapple
1-cup spinach
8 oz. almond coconut milk
3/4 cup frozen peaches
1 frozen banana

Calorie and Nutrition Count

Calories 297
Carbs - 63g
Protein - 3g
Fiber - 4g
Vitamin A - 78mg
Vitamin C - 338mg

Ingredient Spotlight

Goji Berries

Whether you refer to them as wolfberries, Tibetan Goji or Goji berries, this traditionally Asian super food has a lot to offer. They are packed with antioxidants as well as beta-carotene that convert to Vitamin A, so you can't go wrong adding them to your diet. I add them to my smoothie, trail mix and salads in addition to soaking the dried berries (rehydration) to be eaten alone. I've also popped them into an ice cube tray with filtered water and a dash of lemon juice and frozen them. It takes my favorite summertime, homemade lemon-limeade to a whole other level of goodness!

While I'm adding more flavors to my food, I'm also adding fiber (from the seeds) to my diet, more energy, less fatigue and protection from cellular damage. Additionally, Goji berries provide protein from all eight of the essential amino acids the body needs.

Bama Cannon NRG

(Anti-inflammatory, energy, blood purifier)

3 tablespoons ginger
1 baby cucumber
1 frozen banana
1-cup pineapple
1-cup spinach
Juice of 1 lemon
½ cup each of carrot/celery juice/apple (freshly juiced)
½ cup kombucha
Wheatgrass shot (about 1 ounce)
1/8 tsp. kelp

Calorie and Nutrition Count

Calories - 346
Carbs - 97g
Protein - 8g
Fiber - 5g
Vitamin A - 555mg
Vitamin C - 116mg

Ingredient Spotlight

Dark Chocolate

I specified dark chocolate to spotlight; the other variety, namely milk chocolate and cocoa powder, are considered waste products – due to the excessive amount of processing it goes through – without the nutritional benefits to be found in dark chocolate. Not only is dark chocolate delicious – and some would say, addictive – dark chocolate is actually good for diabetics due to the low sugar content, as well as those with high blood pressure.

I know what you're thinking when you read, 'high blood pressure benefits.' You're thinking, "Of course it will bring down your blood pressure. Just the idea that you can have chocolate, of any variety is a relaxing thought, right?"

That may be true, but there is scientific evidence to fortify the claim. Dark chocolate is one of the least processed forms of chocolate and contains flavonoids that improve blood flow. Improving your blood flow means your blood flows through the body more freely and gets where it needs to go (heart, lung, brain, cells) without the impediment caused by high cholesterol (high fatty deposits in your bloodstream that can block the smooth flow of "traffic" in your cells), high fat foods in the diet, which leads to lowered blood pressure.

Dark chocolate also contains antioxidants, which protect you from free radicals and helps to build your immunity. The recommendation for a serving is one ounce, but since it's so delicious, a little more probably won't hurt. What will hurt is if you eat the dark chocolate with a bunch of caramel, marshmallows and other forms of high, non-nutritious forms of sugar. You'll negate the positive effects of dark chocolate before the treat makes it to your mouth. Stick to adding it to your smoothies or consuming solid, dark chocolate on its own.

Berry Banana-Nut Blast

(Bacterial infection protection, memory boost)

1-cup frozen blueberries
½-cup fresh (or frozen) coconut
1 frozen banana
8-10 ounces coconut water

Calorie and Nutrition Count

Calories - 370
Carbs - 63g
Protein - 3g
Fiber - 11g
Vitamin A - 3mg
Vitamin C - 125mg

Ingredient Spotlight

Cloves

Arthritis sufferers will delight in knowing the benefits of adding cloves to your health regimen includes helping reduce inflammation. The pain associated with arthritis leads those who suffer from this debilitating condition to look everywhere for a cure not realizing it's been in the spice rack all along!

Cloves are a powerful antioxidant as well, but to say cloves are effective in a multitude of areas is putting it lightly. You have a cold or the flu, add cloves. You have a tooth ache, soak a cotton ball in clove oil and apply it to your gums. You have indigestion, excessive gas or diarrhea, consume cloves in your diet. Better yet, add the spice to your smoothie to build up your immunity to keep from having to deal with these ailments at all. After all, as the cliché goes, an ounce of prevention is worth a pound of cure.

Tart N Sassy

(Energy, digestion, stress reducer, aphrodisiac, anti-inflammatory)

½-cup fresh beets
1-cup spinach
1 stalk celery
1 thumb-sized piece of ginger (the top half of your thumb)
1 large carrot
3 tamarind pods (presoak in warm water to loosen seeds from the fruit)
½ honey crisp apple
1-cup coconut water

Calorie and Nutrition

Calories - 303
Carbs - 78g
Protein - 6g
Fiber - 17g
Vitamin A - 242mg
Vitamin C - 172mg

Ingredient Spotlight

Mint

Recently, I went to a women's conference where several professional women conducted workshops in their area of expertise. One of the workshop presenters provided everyone with a couple of drops of peppermint oil to "lift" them up for the afternoon workshop. I always knew mint was a mood booster, but the boost I felt after rubbing the oil between my palms and inhaling it through my nostrils was a pleasant reminder. I was instantly revived and that boost is only one of the many benefits associated with having mint in your life. In addition to rejuvenating you for the next phase of your day, mint has proven to be effective in the treatment of asthma and allergies, infertility, digestive and respiratory problems, skin care and even weight loss, in some cases. I was most struck to learn mint (the essential oil) acts as an analgesic for breastfeeding mothers who suffer from nipple sensitivity. There's seemingly no limit to the benefits of adding mint to your diet, whether it's your smoothies, your bath, or your hair care regimen. I love all-purpose ingredients, don't you?

Kappow Morning

(Energy, eye protection, skin enhancer)

Pour 8 oz. near boiling water over one green tea bag for five minutes to allow the catechins to be released. Next, remove tea bag and place cup in the freezer (or add a couple of ice cubes) to cool down while you prepare the rest of the ingredients.

While the tea is cooling, prepare the other ingredients:

1 mango cut in chunks
1-cup frozen peach slices
3 mint sprigs

Calorie and Nutrition Count

Calories - 219
Carbs - 66g
Protein - 4g
Fiber - 9g
Vitamin A - 94mg
Vitamin C - 581mg

Ingredient Spotlight

Green Tea

When it comes to green tea, all you have to decide is what part of your body or ailment you'd like to target. Green tea has been around for centuries because it actually works. Whether you want to use it as a fat burner, or focus on disease prevention, green tea is your "guy." Yes, it is an antioxidant, which puts it in a league of its own in karate chopping free radicals and acting as preventive medicine to certain cancers, such as breast and prostate. Lowering bad cholesterol and increasing good cholesterol are also among the super powers exhibited when you add at least three cups of green tea to your regimen each day. Think three cups are a lot? The easiest way to do it is to swap out soda or sugary drinks for one cup of green tea. And if you're adding at least one of these delicious smoothies to your diet each day, substituting water, milk products or fresh juice from your veggies with a cup of fresh brewed green tea makes it so easy, you'll barely feel like you're making sweeping changes to your lifestyle that you can't keep up with. Give it a try and enjoy the benefits today.

Sunshine Burst

(Lower cholesterol/blood sugar, immunity, accelerate wound healing)

1 frozen banana
1 tbsp. chia seeds
1-cup Swiss chard
½-cup frozen mango
1-cup coconut water

Calorie and Nutrition

Calories - 312
Carbs - 61g
Protein - 6g
Fat- 6g
Fiber - 11g
Vitamin A - 76mg
Vitamin C - 217mg

Ingredient Spotlight

Peanut Butter

One serving of peanut butter is only 2 tablespoons, but those two tablespoons are packed with a plethora of powerful protective products to preserve your heart (See how I did that? The five P's of maintaining a smart heart!) by lowering the bad cholesterol in your body – much like the powers of green tea – and increasing the good cholesterol. It's true, there's fat in peanut butter, but it's the kind of fat your body needs for survival. We're so focused on losing fat that we forget the body actually needs a certain amount of fat to function properly. Vitamins A, D, E and K actually need fat to absorb lycopene and beta-carotene, which protect against heart disease. Some of your vital organs need fat as a protective cushion. So go ahead, add a serving to your smoothie. Dip your carrots in a serving of peanut butter and enjoy them. Better yet, get your favorite apple for dipping, that's my go-to nighttime snack. That's a great combination for your taste buds and your heart.

Watermelon Whimsy

(Aphrodisiac, cancer blocker, cell repair, digestion, muscle soreness relief)

¼ head of small red cabbage
2-cups fresh, sweet watermelon
1 tsp. agave nectar
1 handful parsley
½-cup frozen mixed berries
8 oz. coconut water
1 tsp. apple cider vinegar

Calorie and Nutrition Count

Calories - 308
Carbs - 74g
Protein - 5g
Fiber - 8g
Vitamin A - 107mg
Vitamin C - 374mg

Ingredient Spotlight

Apple cider vinegar

Used as an antiseptic and antibacterial. ACV is used to calm an itchy scalp as well as soothe an upset stomach. Of particular interest to chronic dieters and especially bodybuilders, is ACV's ability to break down protein for use in building and maintaining muscle. There are too many benefits to list here, but I'm sure you get the picture – these days, ACV comes in handy for every part of the body from your head to your toes.

I especially love using ACV as the base for my homemade salad dressings. Instead of being restricted to 2 tablespoons of salad dressing for a sugar-filled serving, I make my own concoction of ½ cup ACV, 2 tablespoons of Dijon mustard, 1 teaspoon agave, 1 teaspoon hot chili pepper sauce, ¼ cup olive oil in a salad dressing mixing jar. It makes enough for two healthy servings and I can double it up to enjoy it on all of my salad instead of just the top layer.

Melodious Mango Mélange

(Digestion, toxin flusher, stress/blood sugar regulator)

1 mango
1-cup pineapple
2 oz. cup aloe vera juice
1-cup chopped fresh cilantro
1 tsp. spirulina
Juice of 2 freshly squeezed limes

Calorie and Nutrition Count

Calories - 335
Carbs - 83g
Protein - 7g
Fiber - 11g
Vitamin A - 245mg
Vitamin C - 367mg

Ingredient Spotlight

Mango

Whenever we think of foods that are good for our eyes, we think of carrots, but mangoes do their fair share to protect our vision as well. Mangoes have antioxidants that ward off degeneration of the eyes as we age, so eat mangoes and add them to your smoothies whenever you find them in season. Take care though, mangoes contain 21g carbs in just one small mango, but the potassium…the potassium they contain is tremendous at 564mg per serving!

Tropi-coco Delight

(High antioxidant, vitamin E regenerator, energy, pH regulator, digestion)

1-cup strawberries
½-cup blueberries
8-10 oz. coconut water
1-cup spinach
1 frozen banana
1 tsp. chia seeds
Juice of ½ fresh lemon
2 tsp. agave nectar

Calorie and Nutrition Count

Calories - 288
Carbs - 64g
Protein - 5g
Fiber - 12g
Vitamin A - 58mg
Vitamin C - 320mg

Ingredient Spotlight

Cucumber

First things first, spend the extra money and buy your cucumbers organic – that way, you can leave the skin on and reap *all* the benefits they have to offer.

Cucumbers have a high water content, which is great for those who have trouble getting in their daily H20 needs. Getting in more water is great for those looking to reduce their weight as well as hydrating the body to keep all the cells, organs and systems in the body functioning properly – as well as the important function of increasing metabolism and a great source of Biotin – one of the all important B Vitamin complex.

Tangy and Smart Heart

(Heart disease prevention, digestion, blood purifier, balance)

8 ounces freshly juiced apple juice
½-cup frozen peaches
1 frozen banana
1 knob of ginger
1 tsp. of chia seeds
1 shot glass-size of wheatgrass juice (or 1 scoop if you use the powdered form)
Juice of 1/2 fresh lemon
1-cup of frozen spinach
½-cup of fresh pineapple
2 ounces filtered water

Calorie and Nutrition Count

Calories - 380
Carbs - 84g
Protein - 8g
Fiber - 10g
Vitamin A - 78mg
Vitamin C- 278mg

Ingredient Spotlight

Spinach

Ladies, do you want to ensure the health of your baby, right from the start of its precious, little life?

Spinach can save the day!

Spinach has over half the recommended daily allowance of folic acid, which is the B vitamin you need to ensure the proper development of your fetus when you get pregnant. Spinach has high amounts of many vitamins that are vital for the proper functioning of our cells and organs, so whenever possible, eat your spinach. When it's added to smoothies, it makes the most beautiful emerald-toned color too!

So Fresh and So Clean Burst

(Folic acid, cellular function, energy, blood sugar regulator, stamina, fertility, sex drive increase)

1 cup Italian parsley (regular parsley is fine too)
2 tsp. of maca powder
1 mango
1 frozen banana
Juice of 1 lime
4 strawberries
1 handful of baby spinach
1 baby cucumber
2 tbsp. of shaved ginger

Calorie and Nutrition Count

Calories - 285
Carbs - 60g
Protein - 5g
Fiber - 12g
Vitamin A - 140mg
Vitamin C - 385mg

Ingredient Spotlight

Limes

Traditionally, limes are inexpensive, but lately, the prices have skyrocketed due to an infection in Mexico -- specifically, the lime trees.

Even though the prices are more than three times the amount they normally would be, depending on what part of the world you live in, the health benefits are worth the price of the limes any day of the week. Why?

Just a couple of reasons are:
For diabetics, limes -- any citrus fruit, really -- have soluble fiber in them that slows down the absorption of carbs. That soluble fiber keeps the blood sugar from spiking.

Other at-risk groups who can benefit from incorporating limes into their life are those who suffer from congestion, such as those who have allergies. The flavonoids in the lime peel are particularly helpful for allergy sufferers.

Carrot Cake Deluxe

(Gas, nausea, fertility, energy, digestion)

2 small carrots
¼ tsp. cinnamon
½ tsp. nutmeg
8 oz. unsweetened vanilla almond milk
1 frozen banana
2 tsp. maca powder
¼-cup chopped walnuts
2 ounces prune juice

Calorie and Nutrition Count

Calories - 467
Carbs - 61g
Protein - 8g
Fat - 24g
Fiber - 12g
Vitamin A - 360mg
Vitamin C - 35mg

Ingredient Spotlight

Cinnamon

Similar to nutmeg, cinnamon can be used for gas and preventing nausea, but the claims that it lowers the blood sugar and is good to treat diabetes have not been supported by substantial research. Cinnamon may not have a bunch of vitamins, but it does have iron and manganese – a mineral that helps make connective tissue in your body.

A side note for the fat grams in the recipe above:

Don't be afraid of this fat, it's good fat. It comes from the Omegas in the almond milk and the walnuts, which are healthy fats. Remember, the body needs fat to absorb vitamins A, C, D, E and K. If you're going to consume fat, healthy fats, such as those from unsaturated fats are ideal.

Fresh Life of PYE

(Digestion, immunity, allergy protection)

¼ medium-sized jicama
¾-cup fresh pineapple
1 handful of cilantro
2 handfuls of spinach (or kale)
1/8 tsp. kelp
1 tsp. spirulina powder
4 ounces fresh squeezed citrus juice
1 banana
1 tsp. chia seeds
6 ounces of filtered or alkaline water
Optional: Add 6 ice cubes

Calorie and Nutrition Count

Calories - 300
Carbs - 66g
Fat - 5g
Fiber - 12g
Protein - 8g
Vitamin C - 148mg
Vitamin A - 182mg

Ingredient Spotlight

Pineapple

This sweet, succulent fruit does double duty. One 4-ounce serving packs enough of a punch to provide your entire day's worth of vitamin C. I also recommend eating pineapple before your meal because it contains an enzyme called bromelain. Bromelain helps your body break down foods you eat in order to help with digestion. Plainly put, this enzyme acts in the same way as a "meat tenderizer" in that it naturally helps break down your foods in order for them to digest easier without destroying the nutrients. Better digestion of your food means the body has the ability to use the nutritional properties of the food and get rid of what you don't need in a more purposeful way. This can also lead to weight loss.

Sparkle, Splash and Fly

(Cellular repair, digestion, energy)

¼ large cucumber
1 handful of fresh spinach
1-cup of freshly juiced carrots/celery
4 sprigs of fresh cilantro
½-cup fresh mango
1 tsp. organic apple cider vinegar
Juice of 1 fresh squeezed lime
1 frozen banana
1/8 tsp. kelp
1 scoop of powdered wheatgrass
10 ounces filtered water

Calorie and Nutrition Count

Calories - 298
Carbs - 69g
Protein - 7g
Fiber - 15g
Vitamin A - 536mg
Vitamin C - 150mg

Ingredient Spotlight

Blueberries

If you are susceptible to bacterial infections, fresh blueberries are just one of the fruits you want to keep handy. They have the uncanny ability to keep bacteria from sticking to the walls of the urinary tract and bladder. Along with cranberries, blueberries also have antioxidant properties that can prohibit cancers, boost your memory and calm an upset stomach.

Geneva's Purple Passion

(Electrolyte restoration)

6 oz. peach Greek yogurt
½-cup frozen blueberries
1 frozen banana
6 oz. unsweetened vanilla almond milk
1 scoop wheatgrass powder (or 1 ounce of chlorophyll)

Calorie and Nutrition Count

Calories - 370
Carbs - 84g
Protein - 18g
Fiber - 8g
Vitamin A - 93mg
Vitamin C - 50mg

Ingredient Spotlight

Potassium

Potassium and sodium are two of the primary minerals that provide electrolytes the body needs for muscle contraction, cellular function, energy and a host of other basic bodily functions essential for daily living.

The potassium in the above recipe has a whopping 644 mg with 192 mg of sodium. This is a good balance of potassium to sodium for proper electrolyte balance as there should be at least a 2:1 ratio of potassium to sodium to maintain a good electrolyte balance.

I made this recipe for my mom who had become dehydrated as a result of the chemotherapy treatments she has to endure for breast cancer. It was high in carbs at 84g, but she needed them for energy as she was completely depleted. This was the first time she actually had no complaints about the taste of this recipe since she still enjoys dairy products and was overjoyed that I used Greek yogurt in this concoction.

Part III
Medium-Carb Smoothie Recipes

One half cup of fruit is typically 15g, 1 slice of toast is 15g, 1 teaspoon of jam = 15g, 8 ounces orange juice = 15g

The above is a typical "quick" breakfast consumed by many. The total is around 60g of carbs. Before the day has begun, if you're a woman, you've already used more carbs than you should per meal. And this isn't even a meal that will satisfy you. Two hours later, you'll be hungry again, guaranteed. Instead prepare your ingredients before bed so you can pop them in the blender while you're preparing to leave for the day. You'll start the day off on much better footing with useful calories to help you get through your morning.

Since the highest amount of carbs per meal for women should be 45g and 60g for men, smoothie recipes in this section range between 46g to 59g. To stay within your target range of carbs per recipe is very easy. Though the smoothie may be delicious, use discipline and split the recipe in half. If you choose make the entire recipe, share with a friend or loved one.

Pineberry Yum Yum

(Digestion, folic acid, anti-inflammatory, bad breath relief)

1-cup frozen peaches
½-cup of freshly juiced celery
1 tsp. fresh lemon juice
4 medium-sized strawberries
1-cup coconut water

Calorie and Nutrition Count:

Total Calories - 195
Protein - 3g
Carbs - 47g
Fiber - 5g
Vitamin A - 19mg
Vitamin C - 545mg

Ingredient Spotlight

Strawberries

Earlier, I shared that my favorite drink, as a youngster, was a strawberry flavored milk drink. As an adult, I couldn't indulge, but I still craved that flavor, so I reinvented a healthy version. I used ½-cup frozen strawberries, 10 ounces of vanilla almond milk, ½-teaspoon of agave and blended. Because the strawberries were slightly tart, I didn't need to add any lemon juice. This drink tasted even better than the strawberry milk drink I loved as a kid. It tasted better and it was now full of nutrients and good fat from the almond milk without the fat from cow's milk I no longer drank.

These delicious buds of goodness deliver 20 percent of the RDA (recommended daily allowance) of vitamin C. The protection provided by vitamin C helps the body repair damaged red blood cells and regenerate vitamin E, one of the body's natural "preservatives."

Smooth n Nutty Pick-Me-Up

(Energy, digestion, fertility, gas relief, weight management, heart health)

1 banana
4 ounces of brewed coffee
4 ounces of unsweetened almond milk
1 tsp. maca powder
Sprinkle cinnamon and nutmeg to taste
2 scoops of cocoa powder
1 tsp. cacao nibs
¼-cup walnuts

Heat the unsweetened almond milk and steep the cacao nibs in the heated milk. Set to the side while you prepare the rest of your ingredients.

Calorie and Nutrition Count

Total Calories - 522
Carbs - 48g
Fat - 30g
Fiber - 12g
Protein - 22g
Vitamin A - 7mg
Vitamin C - 33mg

Ingredient Spotlight

Nutmeg

Nutmeg makes an incredible seasoning, but it's also good at treating gas and bloating. Nutmeg is full of vitamins, including many of the B-complex vitamins (folic acid, niacin and riboflavin) and vitamin C -- which makes it an antioxidant. Using nutmeg means you're including minerals the body needs, such as potassium, manganese, iron and zinc.

And if you have digestion issues, nutmeg can be instrumental in resolving them. It has a history of medicinal use in Indian and Asian cultures.

God's Hooch

(Energy, digestion, wound healing accelerant, cholesterol regulator)

3 broccoli spears
1 frozen banana
½-cup kombucha liquid
1-cup spinach or kale
¼ orange pepper
1 baby cucumber or ¼ regular-sized cucumber
8 ounces freshly juiced apples
Juice of ½ fresh lemon
1 handful fresh cilantro

Calorie and Nutrition Count

Total Calories - 170
Carbs - 46g
Protein - 4g
Fiber - 13g
Vitamin A - 403mg
Vitamin C - 325mg

Ingredient Spotlight

Kale

Kale has a reputation for tasting bitter, but if you blanche it before adding it to your smoothie, it releases the sweet tenderness that will have you coming back for more. Did I mention how one serving provides over 400 percent of the recommended daily value of vitamin K and almost half the vitamin C? This cancer fighting, heart disease preventing, bone-building, sight-saver is all you need to enhance your health and take leaps and bounds towards living younger, longer and prettier!

All Day, All Energy

(Heart health, stamina, mood booster, digestion, muscle cramp relief)

1 frozen banana
¼-cup shredded unsweetened coconut
8 oz. almond coconut milk
1 tsp. maca powder
Sprinkle of fresh nutmeg

Calorie and Nutrition Count

Total Calories - 337
Carbs - 47g
Protein - 8g
Fat - 16g
Fiber - 8g
Vitamin A - 12mg
Vitamin C - 22mg

Ingredient Spotlight

Red Cabbage

The red hue of red cabbage is an automatic green light for the presence of flavonoids, or cancer blocking antioxidants, which reportedly stops cancer growth and repairs cells that have been damaged due to certain cancers.

It also has fiber and even though cabbage is associated with gas and bloating, red cabbage actually helps relieve those symptoms in addition to other digestive ailments, such as irritable bowels and intestinal disorders, such as diverticulitis.

One cup will deliver 85 percent of the recommended daily allowance of Vitamin C, which means your coleslaw is tart, tangy, delicious and packed with disease-fighting phytonutrients designed to protect the body from aging -- or at the very least, dramatically slowing down the process.

Meyerlicious

(Appetite suppressant, anti-inflammatory, bad breath relief, hydration)

1 large carrot
1 medium-sized whole cucumber
1-cup pineapple
1 orange
Juice of 1 Meyer lemon

Calorie and Nutrition Count

Calories - 197
Carbs - 50g
Protein - 6g
Fiber - 8g
Vitamin A - 157mg
Vitamin C - 261mg

Ingredient Spotlight

Oranges

Oranges are good from the outside in as the skin has anti-carcinogenic properties that have passed tests to prevent cervical and breast cancers. The pith (the white part under the skin) is also a source of fiber, which helps lower cholesterol. Then you get to the actual meat of the orange and what do you know? The vitamin C that it's already known for helps to prevent the incidence of gallstones and wrinkles. Just make sure you're getting real orange juice when you decide to drink instead of eat it because many of those cartons of "orange juice" are mostly sugar and only 10 percent or less of the actual fruit.

Krispy G-Pump

(Appetite suppressant, heart disease prevention, energy boost, anti-inflammatory)

1-cup kale
1 baby cucumber (or ¼ regular-sized cucumber)
1 honey crisp apple (or your favorite apple)
2 large carrots
1 handful parsley
2 tbsp. ginger
1 tsp. maca powder
8 oz. green tea

Calorie and Nutrition Count

Calories 198
Carbs - 46g
Protein - 4g
Fiber - 10g
Vitamin A - 570mg
Vitamin C - 182mg

Ingredient Spotlight

Carrots

Everything you've ever heard about carrots is 100 percent true. They *are* good for your eyes, but why and how, you ask?

Carrots provide over 300 percent of the vitamin A you need in your daily diet. That means, your bones get powered packed protection from the beta-carotene that converts to vitamin A and helps build your bones as well as protect your eyesight. Carrots are a natural source of sugar, yet a serving only has eight carbs. The fact that they are such a bright, beautiful shade of orange makes them a cruciferous veggie that's great to improve your mood on a rainy day or any day, for that matter.

Choco-band-a-licious Smoothie

(Mood booster, energy, cancer fighter, bone builder)

1 ½ banana
¼-cup cacao nibs
1 tbsp. agave nectar
1 large kale leaf or spinach
1-inch piece grated ginger
1 tsp. maca powder
1-cup almond coconut milk

Note: Soak the nibs in the cup of almond coconut milk 30 minutes beforehand

Calorie and Nutrition Count

Calories - 335
Carbs - 52g
Protein - 9g
Fat - 15g
Fiber - 15g
Vitamin A - 67mg
Vitamin C - 31mg

Ingredient Spotlight

Cacao Nibs

Study after clinical study reports the benefits of cacao and/or cocoa. Eating real cacao nibs, not the waste product for cacao nibs, i.e. cocoa powder or milk chocolate, drastically reduces the risks for heart attacks due to the magnesium it contains, which actually stabilizes the heart and is responsible for muscle contraction. Eating raw cacao nibs also helps you focus due to a chemical it contains, called phenylethylamanine (PEA). The fiber content compares to eating two servings of broccoli, but you only have to eat an ounce of cacao nibs to get your fiber in. That's why the recipe above has 15g of fiber. The benefits far outweigh the slightly bitter taste of the nibs and since you can soak them in warm almond milk to soften them up and add to your favorite smoothie, there's no reason not to have them on a regular basis…for regularity, get it? The benefits listed here are only a sample of the benefits you'll receive from eating raw cacao. With so many added benefits, what better way is there to satisfy a craving for something sweet? Sweet!

Chock Full O' Veggies

(Breath refresher, blood pressure regulator, appetite suppressant)

1-cup fresh cilantro
½-cup citrus juice mix (see note, pg.11)
½-cup of freshly juiced celery
½-cup of freshly juiced carrots
1-cup spinach
1 baby cucumber (or ¼ regular-sized cucumber)

Calorie and Nutrition Count

Calories - 209
Carbs - 48g
Protein - 7g
Fiber - 7g
Vitamin A - 104mg
Vitamin C - 322mg

Ingredient Spotlight

Celery

Celery tastes saltier than it actually is – with only 35 mg of sodium per 8-inch rib. It's actually good for your blood pressure, according to The Journal of Nutrition. Eating celery stimulates the secretion of bile juice, which leads to a lowering of cholesterol levels. On top of that, if you suffer from constipation, celery is your go-to vegetable because it is chock full of fiber. If you suffer from arthritis, make sure you add lots of chopped celery to your salads as well as the rest of your diet as it also acts as an anti-inflammatory agent due to its ability to remove the uric acid from your system, which is one of the main causes of inflammation.

Street Cred Red

(Aphrodisiac, energy, pH balancer, cellular and connective tissue repair, mood booster)

Brew a cup (8 ounces) of green tea and refrigerate it while you're preparing the rest of your ingredients.

2-cups of watermelon (diced)
1-cup of spinach (chopped)
1 frozen banana
9 sprigs of fresh cilantro
1/8 tsp powdered kelp
Juice of ½ fresh lemon (with pulp)
8 ounces green tea (cooled)

If the banana isn't frozen, quickly peel, slice into chunks and place in the freezer while you're preparing the rest of your ingredients.

Calorie and Nutrition Count

Calories - 227
Carbs - 58g
Protein - 4g
Fiber - 6g
Vitamin A - 120mg
Vitamin C - 128mg

Ingredient Spotlight

Watermelon

We love the juicy sweetness of watermelon. It's especially refreshing on a blazing hot, summer day, but I bet you didn't know watermelon was good for a lackluster libido, did you? Instead of strawberries and chocolate on Valentine's Day, or any romantic night you have planned, chill a cup of watermelon with your champagne and let the fireworks begin!

Watermelon also has an amino acid in it that aids in muscle recovery. Many athletes, as well as those of us who just want to get in better shape, fall off the wagon -- not due to laziness -- but because we know all too well, what the next morning brings; sore muscles that make you feel like you want to roll over and die. This is especially true if you gave it your all during your workout session.

Now you know the delicious secret to muscle recovery: Add a slice of watermelon to your green smoothie or cut a wedge off and eat it straight from the rind. Either way, eat your watermelon within 90 minutes of your tough workout in order to stave off the aches and pains that kill your workout vibe!

Silky Kooky Colada

(Mood booster, energy, digestion, immunity, fertility)

½-cup fresh coconut
1 tsp. vanilla extract
1 frozen banana
3 tsp. maca powder
8-10 ounces unsweetened almond/coconut milk

Calorie and Nutrition Count

Calories - 360
Carbs - 50g
Protein - 5g
Fat - 17g
Fiber - 9g
Vitamin A - 12mg
Vitamin C - 79mg

Ingredient Spotlight

Vanilla

I'd always heard the scent of vanilla was an aphrodisiac, but I thought it was an old wives tale. Turns out, the scent of vanilla actually *is* an aphrodisiac! Using the essential oil versus the extract, which is the most potent form, promotes sexual arousal by stimulating testosterone and estrogen. The next time you're shopping for perfume, notice how many of them contain vanilla. Chemists and smart manufacturers know, in order to compel people to buy, you must appeal to the most basic instinct humans have -- our hormones and sexual appetites. Stimulate people where they are most vulnerable and you're likely to get yourself a sale. Don't believe me? What are the top notes of Passion and White Diamonds -- two of the bestselling perfumes ever? You guessed it – vanilla. It's an unfortunate fact, but it's true.

Vanilla also serves as a powerful stimulant for sleep as well. Try it the next time you're restless, anxious or you just can't seem to settle down to get the zzzz's you need to prepare for the next grueling day. A couple of drops in your rinse cycle or diffused with water and sprayed in the bedroom just before turning out the lights for the night will soon have you sleeping better than you probably have in a long time.

Using the extract form in food, smoothies and nutritional supplements not only improves the flavor and makes you happy due to its mood boosting properties; this wonder spice also has antioxidant properties, which kills free radicals and helps to boost your immune system as well as reported anti-cancer powers.

In short, if you have the opportunity to add vanilla, in any form to your life, don't hesitate; do it tout suite!

Rubberband Smoove (Collagen enhancer)

2 cuties
½ large grapefruit
Juice of 1 lemon
1 inch ginger root piece
Juice of 1 lime
1-cup spinach
1-cup kale

Calorie and Nutrition Count

Calories - 200
Carbs - 56g
Protein - 7g
Fiber - 6g
Vitamin A - 278mg
Vitamin C - 348mg

Ingredient Spotlight

Pears

In addition to being the one fruit with the highest flavor content, pears regulate your bowels like no other. One medium pear has 6 grams of fiber (26 carbs). Six concentrated grams of fiber in one food, not to mention the rest of the food you will most likely consume in a day that contains fiber, is the recipe to release constipation from your life forever. Pears are my number one recommendation – in addition to increasing water consumption – to any client who enjoys the flavor and complains of constipation.

Using a whole pear in your green smoothie is the only fruit you need since it delivers so much flavor, any more sugar will be overkill. The flavor really comes through too; you'll see when you try one of my recipes where pear is the fruit of choice. There are at least five varieties of pears, so experiment with the different varieties until you find the one that works best for you.

Start at the Root

(Aphrodisiac, digestion, heart disease prevention, pH balance)

1 medium-sized carrot
1 small beet (or ½ of a large beet – if it's extra large, use 1/4 beet)
1 small to medium apple
Juice of ½ fresh lemon
4 ounces coconut water

Calories and Nutrition Count

Calories - 189
Carbs - 55g
Protein - 4g
Fiber - 8g
Vitamin A - 149mg
Vitamin C - 27mg

Ingredient Spotlight

Beets

The sweet deliciousness of beets belies their carb content. At only 75 calories and 17 grams of carbs per cup, beets control blood pressure, are said to combat different cancers and contain 3 grams of fiber per serving (1 cup). They are full of folic acid, the B vitamin that helps prevent heart catastrophes, such as heart attacks.

Pregnant women would also do well to incorporate beets in their diet as the folate helps to prevent neural tube defects in the early stages of pregnancy. If you're planning to get pregnant, incorporate beets in your diet well before pregnancy occurs to ensure your baby doesn't suffer from neural tube defects, such as brain malformation or spina bifida – a spinal cord condition that affects the nerves of the spinal cord of the fetus particularly in the first month of pregnancy, which is well before a lot of women even find out they are carrying.

ButterUp! Anti

(Anti-inflammatory, heart health, energy booster, bone protector)

1-cup kale
1-cup pineapple
1 tsp. almond butter
½-cup blueberries
8-10 ounces almond milk

Calories and Nutrition Count

Calories - 342
Carbs - 57g
Protein - 9g
Fat - 12g
Fiber - 7g
Vitamin A - 220mg
Vitamin C- 201mg

Ingredient Spotlight

Grapefruit

Beware that grapefruit contains properties that reportedly interact with certain medications -- negating the effects of certain drugs -- particularly cholesterol lowering medications as well as heart and blood pressure medications. Check with your doctor if you are on any medication to insure you employ a diet that complements your health versus aggravating your condition.

For those who can benefit from adding grapefruit to their diet, high levels of Vitamin C are just one of the benefits of consuming grapefruit besides the natural sweetness of the citrus fruit. There's so much Vitamin C in grapefruit, you only need one half to supply an entire day's worth of this recommended vitamin doing double duty as an antioxidant. I just consumed a whole one, so I've shored up my defenses against strokes and heart disease in addition to helping my skin maintain its elasticity. The only downside is, since I don't like to eat the walls that separate the flesh of the delectable fruit, I've only gotten half the fiber (6 grams total) I could have. Oh well, I guess I'll look to another food source for the rest of the fiber I need!

Healthy Frosty DESSERT

(Mood booster, energy, digestion)

1/3 banana
1-2 tbsp. unsweetened cocoa powder
½ tsp. vanilla
¾-cup almond milk
2-cups ice cubes

Calorie and Nutrition Count

Calories - 272
Carbs - 48g
Protein - 3g
Fat - 3g
Fiber - 3g
Vitamin A - 17mg
Vitamin C - 17mg

Ingredient Spotlight

Grapes

In the summertime, I like to freeze my grapes whole or slice them in half, and freeze them with freshly juiced apples in ice trays with a dash of lemon juice. I will either use them, at some point, in a smoothie, a slushy drink or pop the cube in my mouth for a quick cool down and refresher after my workout session.

Grapes are a great way to combat fatigue and even migraines, not to mention being a great remedy for hangovers. Drink the juice first thing in the morning, or at the onset of a migraine without mixing it with water to get the full benefit and relief as quickly as possible.

A host of other benefits, including protection, prevention and reduction of blood clots, constipation, osteoporosis and bacterial infections result from enjoying a serving of grapes or adding them to your green smoothies.

Happy Day Hangover Relief

(Oxygen enhancer, red blood cell increase, anti-inflammatory, mood booster, electrolyte restoration, breath refresher)

1-cup spinach
½ tsp. ground fresh ginger
¼-cup fresh, chopped cilantro
1 tbsp. chlorophyll
½-cup pineapple
10 ounces coconut water
½-cup seedless grapes (with or without skin)

Calorie and Nutrition Count

Calories - 191
Carbs - 49g
Protein - 2g
Fiber - 3g
Vitamin A - 79mg
Vitamin C - 86mg

Ingredient Spotlight

Coconut Water

The latest craze gaining media attention is coconut water. This highly nutritious fluid that comes from the inside of fresh, young coconuts contains potassium, magnesium and to a lesser degree, sodium and calcium. It's much healthier than the so-called electrolyte-restoring drinks that are loaded with sugar, all in the name of targeting athletes. The best coconuts to retrieve "water" from are no more than nine months old, so it's difficult to truly get the water directly from the coconut unless you live within walking distance of a coconut tree.

Have too much fun partying the night before? Chug a serving (or two) of coconut water before you succumb to the effects of too much alcohol. It's better than chugging water in between alcoholic drinks at the club, which you'll most likely forget to do or abandon during the course of the night. Replenishing lost potassium – a result of dehydration that eventually comes from too much alcohol in the system – is high on the list of things to do to resume normal body functions after a night of pure alcoholic indulgence.

Pina Colada

(Mood booster, energizer, antibacterial, heart health, digestion, cholesterol control)

1-cup fresh chopped spinach
½-frozen banana
½-cup fresh pineapple
1 tsp. coconut oil
¼-cup raw coconut (unsweetened, shredded coconut)
4 ounces coconut water
4 ounces coconut milk

Calorie and Nutrition Count

Calories - 431
Carbs - 57 g
Fat - 24 g
Fiber - 24g
Protein - 4 g
Vitamin A - 65mg
Vitamin C - 76mg

Ingredient Spotlight

Coconut

This is one fat that's good for you! Yay! It relieves stress and who doesn't need stress relief, at some point? Even though coconut is a fat, it's a healthy fat and rather than being bad for weight loss, it's actually so good for weight loss because it helps stimulate your metabolism (i.e. helps your body burn fat).

Coconut also comes in many forms that have so many benefits, it's been called a functional food for its many "functions." Here's a brief description of a few forms of coconut. Some of the following forms listed will be described in further detail throughout this guide.

- Oil – Considered so healthy that it actually helps cholesterol and lowers the chance of heart disease versus all the other oils on the market
- Water – The fluid inside the coconut provides more hydration for your body than regular water and fewer carbs/calories than fruit juice
- Milk – Also great for weight loss due to its fiber content, which is why you feel full after drinking it, which can also keep you from overeating
- Flour – The protein, fiber and fat fill you up and guess what else? It's gluten free! Cooking muffins and baked goods for those suffering from celiac disease becomes much easier to do
- Sugar – This form of sweetener is an especially great resource for diabetics as it has a lower carb count (4g per serving) than any other sweetener on the market

Zesty Life

(Anti-inflammatory, bone-builder, muscle contraction, digestion, pH balance restoration)

1 medium-sized carrot
1 inch piece of ginger
1 Mango
1 small clementine
1-cup cilantro
2 tsp. fresh squeezed lemon juice

Calorie and Nutrition Count

Calories - 223
Carbs - 57g
Protein - 3g
Fiber - 7g
Vitamin A - 201mg
Vitamin C - 210mg

Ingredient Spotlight

Agave Nectar

It's one of nature's sweeteners as it a product of the agave plant. The best advice is to taste your food or drink as you're preparing it to ensure you aren't adding unnecessary amounts of the sweetener out of habit. One serving (1tablespoon) of agave adds 16 carbs, which is still less than table sugar. Agave has gained the reputation for being a great substitute for table sugar due to the fact that you only need about 1/3 as much of it for flavoring versus the amount that would be used for table sugar. Another great benefit of using agave – it dissolves so much easier in cool drinks, which means your iced tea and lemonade get the benefit of this delicious, low-glycemic sweetener without the clump of honey that doesn't dissolve as easy in cool drinks or the sugar crystals from table sugar that settle at the bottom of the glass if not mixed thoroughly.

Sweet Baby Jeeter

(Folate, energy, toxin flusher, menstrual cramp relief, digestion, pH balance)

½ jicama
1 small beet
1 medium-sized carrot
Juice of 1 fresh lemon

Calorie and Nutrition Count

Calories - 216
Carbs - 51
Protein - 5g
Fiber - 22g
Vitamin A - 176mg
Vitamin C - 173mg

Ingredient Spotlight

Jicama

Jicama is a low calorie, root vegetable that can help you manage your weight by curbing your cravings. Ironically, foods high in starch are normally not recommended for diabetics, but Jicama is an exception to this rule. The fiber content of jicama means that it doesn't break down into sugar the body uses and converts to energy right away, which means it can be enjoyed by diabetics without fear of sending blood sugar levels into the stratosphere the way simple, or refined sugars are known to do.

Nu-Bannut Dunk

(Energy boost, focus, digestion)

¼-cup cacao nibs
1 frozen banana
½-cup shredded (unsweetened) coconut
1 tsp. vanilla bean extract
8 ounces almond coconut milk

Calorie and Nutrition Count

Calories - 484
Carbs - 48g
Protein - 8g
Fat - 30g
Fiber - 17g
Vitamin A - 11mg
Vitamin C - 16mg

Ingredient Spotlight

Sweet Potatoes

For a long time, I resisted eating sweet potatoes. I didn't have to resist them very often, as they were only popular during Thanksgiving and Christmas. Nowadays, sweet potatoes are popping up everywhere as a healthier alternative to white potatoes. I must admit I finally gave in after baking them in the oven and flavoring them with a teaspoon of coconut oil. Many other people flavor sweet potatoes with a lot of added ingredients, such as lemon juice, nutmeg, vanilla extract, cinnamon and sugar. All of those ingredients are wonderful and healthy, but to me, the sweet potato has a lot of flavor on its own and I really didn't need anything else.

Now that I've discovered how much I like sweet potatoes, I've also discovered they are a great source of B, C and D vitamins, in addition to iron, magnesium and potassium. Sweet potatoes are another great food for diabetics as they have a low glycemic index and release sugars into the bloodstream at a slower rate than white potatoes.

The Snap Back

(Cellular function, pH balance, energy, digestion)

9 Sprigs fresh cilantro
¼-cup lemon juice
1-cup pineapple
¼ small beet
1 tsp. agave nectar
1½-cup spinach
8 ounces apple/celery/carrot freshly juiced

Calorie and Nutrition Count

Calories - 333
Carbs - 48g
Protein -3g
Fiber - 6g
Vitamin A - 114mg
Vitamin C - 276mg

Ingredient Spotlight

Chia Seeds

The fact of the matter is there will never be a world we live in where everyone eats a plant-based diet primarily. We just have to get used to that fact; especially as B12 is mainly sourced from animal protein (in addition to legumes) and we need our B12 to function. It's one vitamin our bodies use to absorb and convert the nutrients in our food to energy.

The next best thing is to work to incorporate as much plant-based nutrition into the diet as possible. Chia seeds are power packed with protein and the type of fat your body needs to function in addition to a host of healthful benefits, such as helping to control your blood pressure and your digestive system. Chia seeds get a lot of press for weight loss because once they are soaked in liquid, they expand. When you eat them, you have a full sensation in your belly for an extended amount of time.

Before I transitioned to an 80 percent plant-based diet, I began to add chia seeds into my beef stew instead of adding flour to thicken it. I loved it! Now, I add them to many of my smoothie recipes when I want to make sherbet or popsicles. Sometimes, when I get a taste for some chocolate pudding, mixing almond or coconut milk with a frozen banana, vanilla extract, a few cacao nibs, a scoop of cocoa powder and a sprinkle of chia seeds is all it takes for me to enjoy my very own "Jell-O" pudding. It freezes great to make the kids a chocolate pudding pop, too.

Part IV
Low-Carb Smoothie Recipes

All of the smoothie recipes in this section fall into the category of low-carb since they are below the target for a woman (45g) per meal. You'll find the recipes are just as delicious, if not more so than those with higher carb counts. The difference is, by now, you've trained your taste buds; you've begun to practice discipline; and you've opened your mind to the idea that low-carb does not equal "low" or "disgusting" taste where green smoothies are concerned. The recipes yield at least 16 ounces, if not more of delicious smoothie. You get full, and you're naturally helping your body detox itself -- as it is already built to do -- by feeding it good, whole, healthy food. That's all you have to do–treat your body good and it will return the favor.

Peaches and Greenery

(Immunity, menstrual cramp relief, anti-aging, acid reflux relief, energy)

½-cup frozen peaches
Juice of 1 fresh lemon
2-cups Romaine lettuce
½ banana
½ clove of garlic
1 small (peeled, if not organic) cucumber
½-cup spinach
10 ounces aloe Vera juice

Calorie and Nutrition Count

Total Calories - 94
Protein - 1g
Carbs - 18g
Fiber - 4g
Vitamin A - 134 mg
Vitamin C - 130mg

Ingredient Spotlight

Peaches

One serving of peaches is a juicy, delicious way to get in 1/5 of the daily recommendation of retinol, or vitamin A. Your eyes will thank you since vitamin A helps you see better - especially in the dark. If you're pregnant, getting in your vitamin A helps with the development of your baby as well as forming red blood cells. And let's not overlook the vitamin C content. One cup of juicy peaches has 280mg of vitamin C, also known as the antioxidant that combats damage to your cells, helps to produce collagen and also helps your body heal wounds, cuts and bruises.

Pineapple Spice

(Immunity, blood pressure regulator, red blood cell enhancer)

1 frozen banana cut into chunks
2 large leaves of Swiss chard
2-inch piece of ginger
½-cup of fresh pineapple chunks
½-cup of tamarind juice
1 organic baby cucumber (If you don't buy organic, peel it, as it can contain pesticides)
½-cup cilantro or parsley

Calorie and Nutrition Count

Calories - 167
Carbs - 43g
Protein - 3g
Fiber - 11g
Vitamin A - 96mg
Vitamin C - 163mg

Ingredient Spotlight

Parsley

Parsley may be known for its breath enhancing properties, but it's also good for lowering the bad cholesterol levels in your body. Added to that, the vitamin K in parsley helps to build your bone density – something those at risk for falls and potential bone fractures will appreciate immensely. It contains zero carbs, so feel free to add it to your smoothies with abandon as well as using it in your salads and on baked potatoes. The antioxidants it contains provide smart heart protection as well properties that help to purify your blood.

Goddess of Green Beauty

(Skin/hair health, thyroid regulator, blood sugar regulator, pH balance)

2 broccoli spears
1-cup fresh chunks of jicama
½ of fresh lemon
1 baby cucumber
½ banana
½-cup fresh pineapple
2 tamarind pods (soaked in hot water and seeds removed)
1/8 tsp. kelp
1 tsp. spirulina powder

Calorie and Nutrition Count

Calories - 111
Carbs - 27g
Protein - 3g
Fiber - 12g
Vitamin A - 89mg
Vitamin C - 140mg

Ingredient Spotlight

Broccoli

This super food is filled with life enhancing vitamins like vitamin C, Calcium, vitamin A, fiber and even five grams of protein in one serving. Broccoli is good for so many things, there isn't enough space here, but you can look forward to a reduction in the risk of developing cataracts, prevention of prostate issues, a reduction in the risk of bladder *and* colon cancer, as well as a 50 percent reduction in the risk of developing heart disease. Broccoli is a staple everyone needs to utilize in the kitchen, and – prepared properly (steaming is best) – it tastes simply delicious! Don't overcook it. All the life enhancing benefits will simply die if you do.

Chi-Chi Splash

(Electrolyte balance, anti-inflammatory, eyesight protector)

2 leaves chopped Swiss chard
1/3 cup red cabbage
1-cup fresh pineapple
1 tsp. chia seeds
1/3 piece large cucumber
½-cup fresh tamarind juice

Calorie and Nutrition Count

Calories - 197
Carbs - 40g
Protein - 8g
Fat -5g
Fiber - 11g
Vitamin C - 217mg
Vitamin A - 133mg

Ingredient Spotlight

Cabbage

There is a compound in cabbage that can stop skin, breast and prostate cancer in their tracks! Not only that, cabbage can also lower the risk of bladder cancer, stroke, cataracts and heart disease. One great way to ensure that you get all the benefits of cabbage is to make sure you don't overcook it. Lightly steam it and enjoy – or better yet – put some cabbage in your smoothie and slurp 'til your heart is content.

The Best of All Worlds

(Diuretic, blood pressure regulator, anti-inflammatory, digestion, blood purifier)

1 granny smith apple
1 grapefruit
1 rib of celery
1 one-inch piece ginger root
2 leaves of mint
1 shot of freshly juiced wheatgrass

Calorie and Nutrition Count

Calories - 113
Carbs - 27g
Protein - 6g
Fiber - 9g
Vitamin A - 60mg
Vitamin C - 79mg

Ingredient Spotlight

Bananas

More than just a great source of potassium – bananas provide a healthy source of energy that can satisfy your sweet tooth at the same time they help your body recover after a great workout. Bananas also contain chromium, which enhances the effects of insulin and helps metabolize fat; and if you have heartburn, reach for a banana before an antacid as the enzymes in bananas act as a natural antacid.

If you've ever had a digestive problem and suffer from constipation, here's your non-pharmaceutical remedy. They're also known to provide potassium, and if you ever run low on potassium, your body will certainly let you know. Leg cramps is a sign of low potassium levels. A banana per day will help keep leg *and* foot cramps away.

When used in your smoothies, bananas serve as a non-artificial thickening-agent; that way, you don't have to use xanthan gum, Irish moss or even dairy products if you're moving towards a vegan lifestyle.

Once you become accustomed to the taste, if you don't care for bananas, all you taste is the deliciousness of your concoction. As a former banana-hater, I guarantee it.

Splendor in the Grass

(Immunity, red blood cell enhancer, joint pain relief, pH balance)

Juice of 1 Meyer lemon
½-cup fresh pineapple
¼-cup freshly chopped cilantro
1/3 large cucumber
4 ounces aloe vera juice
1 tsp. freshly grated ginger
1-cup fresh spinach
2 ounces fresh wheatgrass juice

Calorie and Nutrition Count

Calories - 101
Carbs - 20g
Protein - 4g
Fiber - 4g
Vitamin A - 148mg
Vitamin C - 108mg

Ingredient Spotlight

Ginger

There's absolutely no fat in ginger and although it's spicy to the palate, it is soothing to an upset stomach and a host of other ailments. Ginger helps prevent heart disease and stroke as well as preventing cancer cells from multiplying. Ginger fights inflammation as well as bacteria, which can cut down on visits to the doctor if you're prone to infections. Many that suffer from arthritis find relief in ginger, whether it's taken straight, or mixed in with tea or your favorite spicy, Indian dish.

Special note: When adding ginger to your smoothies, use a cheese grater or microplane to shred the ginger, if you aren't putting it in the juicer. Grating the ginger makes the tough, fibrous strands available for absorption in the body in order to use all the wonderful nutrients ginger contains.

Native Earth Elixir

(Energy, immunity, digestion, red blood cell enhancer)

1-cup spinach
1 baby cucumber
1 avocado
¼-cup freshly chopped cilantro
2 ounces freshly juiced wheatgrass
1-cup frozen peach slices
8 ounces kombucha

Calorie and Nutrition Count

Calories - 175
Carbs - 28g
Protein - 6g
Fiber - 6g
Vitamin A - 161mg
Vitamin C - 332mg

Ingredient Spotlight

Kombucha

The Mayo Clinic defines kombucha tea as a fermented drink made with yeast, sugar, black, green or white tea, vinegar and bacteria cultures. Kombucha tea kept chilled, or at room temperature is said to provide probiotic (bacteria the body needs to maintain a healthy balance for good digestion) benefits and is comparable to capsules and powders found in health food stores.

Fermented foods are a godsend especially to the plant-based society because they contain B vitamins that are normally only found in meat products. That's another reason kombucha has found its way into the mainstream after being an ancient Chinese secret for hundreds of years. Any food product that gives you energy will be welcomed by society-at-large as we all seem to be energy-starved at some point during the day. Consider swapping out your afternoon cup of java for a refreshing drink of kombucha. Not only will you help break your body's dependency on caffeine, you'll be glad for a natural burst of energy that does double duty by providing healthy bacteria the body needs to stave off infection and build the immune system.

Garden of Eden Smoothie

(Energy, digestion, breath refresher, pH balance, immunity, decongestant, acid reflux relief)

1 packed cup Swiss chard
1 tsp. fresh lemon juice
1 frozen banana
1 handful cilantro

Calories and Nutrition

Calories - 133
Carbs - 43 g
Fiber - 4g
Protein - 6g
Vitamin A - 66mg
Vitamin C - 83mg

Ingredient Spotlight

Flax

One indisputable fact about flax is that it ***is*** your friend. Why, you ask? Flax contains essential fatty acids our body needs, but can't make on our own. We have to get it from outside sources like flax. Flax contains omega-3 fatty acids that we simply don't get enough of in our diet. Omega-3's are found mostly in fish and they have a reputation for preventing certain cancers, such as breast and endometrial cancers due to their ability to block estrogen absorption. It may not add flavor, but adding flax to your diet will definitely add a boost to your digestive system as the insoluble fiber helps to relieve constipation and keep you regular.

Float Like a Butterfly

(Folate, anti-inflammatory, metabolism booster, weight management)

2-cups chopped baby spinach
1 pear
½-cup strawberries
Juice of 1 lime
1-inch piece ginger
1 tsp. of bee pollen

Calorie and Nutrition Count

Calories - 163
Carbs - 28g
Protein - 4g
Fiber - 8g
Vitamin A - 114mg
Vitamin C - 39mg

Ingredient Spotlight

Bee Pollen

If you're allergic to bees, this probably isn't an ingredient you want to use in your green smoothies. I can't vouch for the effects, but I've read that you have the potential to suffer some of the same effects from ingesting bee pollen that you would endure if a bee stung you.

For those who aren't allergic, bee pollen has amino acids and enzymes that help every cell in the body, including the largest organ in the body -- the skin. For acne sufferers, bee pollen has enzyme properties that heal wounds, including acne, eczema, rashes and even hives.

Adding the powder to your favorite smoothie not only provides a nutty flavor, depending on the strength used, it acts as a fat flusher, detoxifier and weight loss aid that's low in calories and provides a nice energy boost as it is a great source of B12 vitamins.

Nutri-Treat Smoothie

(Allergy relief, energy, weight management)

1-cup frozen mixed berries
¼-cup coconut
½-cup pineapple
1-cup spinach
1 tsp. bee pollen
8 ounces coconut water

Calorie and Nutrition Count

Calories - 264
Carbs - 37g
Protein - 6g
Fat - 11g
Fiber - 11g
Vitamin A - 5
Vitamin C - 112

Special note: One simple change can affect the entire nutrition profile. Changing the spinach preparation from boiled with salt to fresh, organic baby spinach reduced the vitamin A content from 381 mg to 5 mg, the calorie count reduced by 31, the protein reduced by 4, the vitamin C from 141 to 96 and the sodium, a whopping 647 mg reduced to 96 after changing the prep for the spinach. Little changes make a big difference.

Ingredient Spotlight

Blackberries

If you suffer during allergy season, you definitely want to add blackberries to your smoothies, fruit cups and awesome homemade fruit cubes (drop one berry per cube section and fill with water before freezing). Blackberries contain Quercetin – a compound that acts as an antihistamine. Allergy sufferers will find this useful – especially during the summer months when hay runs amok in the atmosphere.

Choco-Cherry Dreams

(Insomnia relief, anti-anxiety)

1-cup pitted cherries
8-10 oz. almond coconut milk
¼-cup fresh coconut (shredded, unsweetened)
1 tsp. vanilla extract
1 tsp. valerian root extract

Calorie and Nutrition Count

Calories - 205
Carbs - 25g
Protein - 3g
Fat - 11g
Fiber - 5g
Vitamin A - 11mg
Vitamin C - 15mg

Ingredient Spotlight

Cherries

If you suffer from arthritis, or have inflammation and pain in your joints, cherries just may provide the relief you seek. They are also a great snack to have before going to bed to help you get a good night of sleep. They are packed with antioxidants as well, and the sweet tart flavor makes for some of the best tasting smoothies ever.

Rainier cherries happen to be my favorite cherry, appropriately so given that I seem to love the most expensive "anything" available. While cherries are arguably one of the most expensive fruits around, Rainier cherries have to take the proverbial cake. When they are in season, I've personally paid as much as $6.99 per pound for the luscious, succulent fruit. They are only in season during the hottest months of the year (late June through August), so it stands to reason, you would have to pay premium prices to enjoy them.

I will never forget the first time I tasted them and fell in love with them. I worked in a doctor's office and one of the physicians brought his "fruit of the month" box of cherries in to share with the staff. Discovering the health benefits in addition to the delicious taste and expense of these premium cherries takes the term, "good bedside manner" to a whole new level of wonderful.

Chocolate Cream Supreme

(Folate, energy, heart health)

1 frozen banana
½ avocado
1 tsp. cocoa powder
10 oz. almond coconut milk
1 tsp. coconut

Calorie and Nutrition Count

Calories - 252
Carbs - 32g
Protein - 4g
Fiber - 8g
Vitamin A - 14mg
Vitamin C - 22mg
Fat - 12g

Ingredient Spotlight

Avocado

They are one of the best fats around that protect the heart from heart disease and also have the ability to lower cholesterol. If you want to ensure your skin stays smooth and supple, gobble up some avocado! The good fat in avocado actually helps your skin stay youthful and provides elasticity to keep 'em guessing when they're trying to figure out your age. It's also one of the few fruits that are actually low in sugar, so you don't have to worry about sending your blood sugar through the roof with a single serving, thank goodness.

Sweet n Spicy Goodness

(Heart health, bacterial growth protection, pH balance, joint pain relief)

2-cups cilantro
1-cup frozen peaches
Juice of 1 fresh lemon
1-cup unsweetened cranberry juice
½-cup pineapple
1 tsp. grated ginger

Calorie and Nutrition Count

Total Calories - 120
Carbs - 29g
Protein - 5g
Fiber - 3g
Vitamin A - 16mg
Vitamin C - 460mg

Ingredient Spotlight

Cilantro

Cilantro is a great source of vitamin K, which helps your blood clot. Vitamin K is also a fat-soluble vitamin, which means you need to eat fat (good fat) in order for it to be absorbed. Choosing cilantro leaves that are dark green in color means they contain higher amounts of chlorophyll, which has been reported to build immunity. Staving off a seasonal cold or the flu has me stuffing my smoothies with as much cilantro as I can fit in the jar.

It's also good to have on hand for stomach discomfort and did I mention how easy it is to grow? Cilantro gave me a boost as one of the very first herbs I planted that didn't die when I first became interested in gardening.

Italian Juice Smoothie (Homemade Tomato Juice)

(Prostate protection, hearth health, blood pressure reducer, pH balance, overall health)

1 pint of grape tomatoes
1 finely chopped clove of garlic
1 tsp. Worcestershire sauce
1/8 tsp ground pepper
Juice of 1 freshly squeezed lemon
2 tbsp. ACV or balsamic vinegar
1 rib of celery
1 pinch kosher salt

Calorie and Nutrition Count

Calories - 114
Carbs - 27g
Protein - 4g
Fiber - 7g
Vitamin A - 84mg
Vitamin C - 171mg

Ingredient Spotlight

Tomatoes

The sweet taste of grape tomatoes takes a salad to new heights, but all varieties of tomatoes have something special to offer. Men should eat tomatoes like there is no tomorrow as tomatoes lower the risk of prostate cancer by as much as 40 percent!

Tomatoes and tomato products help lower bad cholesterol and stave off heart disease, which is due to lycopene. Men may be the targets of prostate disease, but lycopene is an antioxidant that is also reported to stave off colon and cervical cancer as well as lung, stomach and breast cancer.

Ginger Kale Ade

(Anti-inflammatory, digestion, energy, heart health, overall wellness)

1 thumb-sized piece of ginger
2-cups kale
2 tbsp. fresh lemon juice
1 granny smith apple
10 ounces coconut water

Calorie and Nutrition

Calories - 190
Carbs - 43g
Protein - 4g
Fiber - 6g
Vitamin A - 413mg
Vitamin C - 378mg

Ingredient Spotlight

Lemon

Lemons have so many benefits – I'm going to focus on a couple that I have found to be most significant in my life and those closest to me. Although they aren't green, lemons help restore the body's pH balance, which is essential for proper function in every cell of your body. Like wheatgrass, lemons act as a blood purifier, helping to restore the body to an optimal level of being.

When you add lemon to your daily regimen, notice how much better your digestion becomes. Seriously, pay attention to your body and note how much more energy you have as a result of regular bowel movements. Lemons actually help digestion by causing your intestines to contract and move waste along and out of your system instead of being stuck and causing you to feel bloated and sluggish. Trust me when I tell you, a "well-oiled" digestive system is the next best thing to…I don't know, arriving at the perfect weight, getting an unexpected raise, a phone call from your favorite person…all of the above. Try adding lemons to your daily regimen -- you'll see.

Serving Suggestion: First thing in the morning, drink a cup of warm water with the juice of half a fresh lemon in it before you start your day. Everyday.

3 CCs (Celery, Cucumber, Coconut Water)

(Joint pain/allergy relief, anti-inflammatory, tumor blocker, blood pressure regulator)

1-cup coconut water
½ cucumber
1-cup pineapple
2 tbsp. ginger
Juice of 1 lime
2 celery ribs

Calorie and Nutrition Count

Calories - 158
Carbs - 39g
Protein - 3g
Fiber - 4g
Vitamin A - 10mg
Vitamin C - 223mg

Ingredient Spotlight

Cranberry

I've loved the tart taste of cranberry juice since I was a kid, but I had no idea it was protecting me from bacteria build up and possible kidney infections. The proanthocyanidins found in the tart berry keep bacteria from sticking to the sides of your bladder, making it near impossible for bad bacteria to build up and multiply, causing the pain and discomfort indicative of a urinary tract or kidney infection. You only enjoy the benefits to prevent infection, not cure infection.

Added to that, the same compound that prevents bacteria from clinging to the walls of your bladder, acts in much the same way for your teeth. Yep! Consuming cranberries on a regular basis has the ability to stop bacteria growth on your teeth too.

And, if you've got the flu, a cold, or even an ulcer, make sure you stock up on cranberries – the juice or the berries themselves. Caution though: if you decide to consume the juice, check the sugar content as sugar causes cavities and can cancel out the good benefits of cranberries if there's too much sugar in the juice.

Napa or Bust

(Digestion, cholesterol control, allergen relief, eyesight protectant)

Juice of 1 fresh lime
¼-cup fennel
1 small avocado
1-cup pineapple
8-10 ounces coconut water

Calorie and Nutrition Count

Calories -191
Carbs - 39g
Protein - 4g
Fat - 21g
Fiber - 3g
Vitamin A - 5mg
Vitamin C - 208mg

Ingredient Spotlight

Apricots

Vitamins A and C plus 3 grams of fiber in one serving – the tiny looking apricot packs a wallop and provides much needed antioxidant protection for optimal cellular function in the body. Potassium, however, is the real star of the show when it comes to this juicy, year-round treat. One serving of raw apricots (1 cup) contains 427 mg potassium! That's more than a banana (422mg). The dried variety commonly used in trail mix contains even more at 514mg per ½ cup serving.

Who knew?

What's the big deal about potassium, you ask? Simply put, potassium is the be all and end all of cellular function in the body. Without it, you can't build muscle; your body can't break down carbs and use them for energy, and you need potassium for proper cardiac function. Sounds like a plan to add a cup of apricots (freeze the dried ones for a tart, refreshing treat) to your regimen as often as you can.

Clara's Cleanse

(Heart health, arthritis relief, pH balance,
cholesterol control, immunity)

1 clove of finely chopped garlic
1 beet (blanch, chop and use the 8 ounce of the water to mix this smoothie)
1-cup cilantro
3 tsp. ginger
Juice of 1 fresh lemon

Calorie and Nutrition Count

Calories - 71
Carbs - 23g
Protein - 3g
Fiber - 3g
Vitamin A - 51mg
Vitamin C - 31mg

Ingredient Spotlight

Honey

It tastes delicious, it's nutritious and used sparingly, yet effectively, honey can be your best friend.

There are so many reports in the media lately giving honey a bad rap; calling it nothing but another form of sugar that we'd do well to stay clear of, but one thing is missing from those reports: the fact that moderation is the key. Sure, if you use an excessive amount of anything, the benefits will be reduced, so let's take a look at the good aspects of honey that far outweigh the overblown reports in the news.

Honey is used as an antiseptic, antibacterial and antioxidant, but a little publicized fact about honey is; it stimulates the growth of good bacteria – probiotics – in your gut. Therefore, it's considered a prebiotic, which is of supreme importance to helping the body ward off infection and build immunity to keep you from getting sick due to infections or other nasty ailments that want to take over your body. If ever you have to take antibiotics to cure an infection, be sure to sparingly incorporate the raw, unfiltered variety into your smoothies or other parts of your diet. You'll be able to enjoy all of the nutritional benefits and get back on your feet a lot sooner with less chances of having to endure the side effects that can come with taking antibiotics.

Greench Butternut Operator

(Digestion, energy, heart health, focus)

1 tsp. almond butter
1 small avocado
1/3-cup cacao nibs
1 scoop dark chocolate cocoa powder
8 ounces vanilla almond milk
1 tsp. vanilla extract

Calorie and Nutrition Count

Calories 437
Carbs - 43g
Protein - 16g
Fat - 43g
Fiber - 16g
Vitamin A - 13mg
Vitamin C - 39mg

Ingredient Spotlight

Coffee

Warning! Everyone can't tolerate coffee in order to enjoy its many benefits. I happen to be among those who can't as it instantly cramps up my stomach and gives me digestive complications. Maybe that was too much information for you, but I wanted to illustrate that everyone simply can't tolerate all foods. That's why I've worked really hard to come up with a lot of different combinations for you to try as you move toward your own *Green Smoothie Bliss*.

Coffee is a natural diuretic and a naturally caffeinated product made from different coffee beans grown around the world. At 85mg per 8 ounce cup, the caffeine found in coffee really is marginal when compared to other sources of caffeinated drinks, such as some energy drinks where the amount of caffeine is triple that found in one serving of coffee.

The health benefits related to coffee stem from the amounts of potassium and magnesium found in a serving of coffee, which are two minerals the body needs for cardiovascular function, muscle contraction and cellular growth are the mainstays in a serving of coffee. As long as you aren't consuming 10 cups of coffee on a daily basis, there's no harm, no foul to enjoying your java and don't let anyone tell you different.

Sunset Healing Bliss

(Anti-inflammatory, cancer growth/spread inhibitor, antibacterial, antifungal, blood sugar regulator, eyesight protectant, pH balance, heart health, bone protector)

1 orange
1 medium-sized carrot
2-inch piece of ginger
8 ounces of turmeric tea (or 1 teaspoon of turmeric powder)

Calories and Nutrition Count

Calories - 136
Carbs - 32g
Protein - 3g
Fiber - 6g
Vitamin A - 154mg
Vitamin C - 149mg

Ingredient Spotlight

Turmeric

Curcumin, the active substance in turmeric, has so many benefits, I could write a booklet on this one spice by itself.

Particularly good for those with heartburn and other digestive problems as well as inflammation, turmeric is the spice for you if you've been afflicted with arthritis, heart disease, or osteoarthritis among a host of other diseases and ailments. Diabetics should take care when using turmeric though. The glycemic index-reducing effects can be so potent that if you're already taking medication to treat diabetes, your blood sugar levels may dip below what is considered healthy.

As a popular spice in Indian dishes, turmeric, or curry powder, adds a spicy flavor that can be mild or highly spicy depending on your preference. I love to add it to dips, my homemade hummus recipes and even when I'm making my favorite bean dish. Knowing that I'm adding an exotic flavor while keeping my blood sugar levels in check keeps me happy as well as my doctor. You gotta love that!

Apple CinnaSwirl

(Digestion, energy, gas relief, mood booster)

6 ounces freshly juiced apple juice
4 ounces almond milk
2 ounces coconut milk
½-frozen banana
Sprinkle of cinnamon
Sprinkle of nutmeg

Calories and Nutrition Count

Calories - 248
Carbs - 35g
Protein - 2g
Fat - 4g
Fiber - 5g
Vitamin A - 10mg
Vitamin C - 19mg

Ingredient Spotlight

Blackstrap Molasses

I know, I know, blackstrap molasses has been referred to as nothing but refined table sugar, but that is far, far from accurate.

Blackstrap molasses has been boiled three times to reduce it to its purest form and the minerals it contains put this in a category all on its own, well not entirely on its own as it does fall into the super food category.

I use it in my baked beans recipe, and yes, people have reported feeling much happier after they've had my baked beans. Until I began to research how food affects the body, I had no idea blackstrap molasses was a mood booster!

BSM is also the good culprit when it comes to improving anemia and even muscle cramps and spasms, according the National Institute of Health.

Calcium, one of the fifteen minerals essential for proper cellular function, is a component of BSM and thus provides a host of benefits similar to, and in many cases better than, the cow secretions, such as milk and yogurt, the human species could do just fine without -- in my opinion -- as the human race is the only species that consumes the milk of another species for its health and wellbeing.

Skin conditions, such as acne, psoriasis and eczema, in addition to signs of premature aging, such as wrinkles are all benefits you'll receive by adding BSM to your green smoothie.

South of the Border Nectar

(Eyesight protectant, weight management, digestion, cholesterol control)

2 nectarines
6 ounces freshly squeezed apple juice
4 ounces tamarind juice
Sprinkle of nutmeg
8 ounces alkaline water (8-9.5 pH)

Calorie and Nutrition Count

Calories - 177
Carbs - 42g
Protein - 2g
Fiber - 3g
Vitamin A - 13mg
Vitamin C - 45mg

Ingredient Spotlight

Tamarind Fruit

Ah, the tamarind fruit -- this is my holy grail of tart fruit. I tried not to use it in too many recipes, but really, I am in love with this fruit and you will be too, if you like tart flavors. If you can believe it, tamarind is just as tart as lemon -- perhaps even more -- and the holistic effects on the body are reason enough for you to experience this little-known fruit for yourself.

I've been working with tamarind for about three years simply because I love the flavor, but I've only recently discovered the metabolism boosting, weight loss effects of this Mexican, Asian and African fruit. Discovering this information only increased its value to me. It may be a challenge to release the pulp from the seed, but the reward will be worth your hard work. I recommend soaking the pods in just enough warm water to cover the pods a couple of hours prior to using in your smoothie; this way, you don't have to drain the water -- you can use the water as the liquid base in your smoothie.

I actually discovered tamarind, also known as garcinia cambogia, in the Latino grocery store and have since become obsessed with finding it in different varieties. It makes a wonderful addition to my smoothie recipes as well as cooking. This fruit also has antibacterial properties as well as reducing bad cholesterol levels in the body.

Godiva Aura

(Digestion, skin enhancer, blood pressure regulator, mood booster)

1 carrot
1 pear
2 ribs of celery
2-cups Romaine lettuce
2 mint leaves
Juice of 1 fresh lemon (or 2 Tablespoons lemon juice from bottle)

Calorie and Nutrition Count

Calories - 157
Carbs - 32g
Protein - 1g
Fiber - 14g
Vitamin A - 408mg
Vitamin C - 32mg

Ingredient Spotlight

Nectarines

One of my trade secrets of making a delightfully tart and tasty peach cobbler is actually using nectarines in the recipe along with peaches. No one has ever asked because the two fruits are so similar, you can barely tell the difference. I certainly can because I love tart and tangy flavors and to me, nectarines are more tart than peaches.

Aside from the flavor, nectarines are one of the best fruits to add to your diet if you're trying to lose weight *and* you have a sweet tooth. A medium nectarine has only 15grams of carbs, so it's a perfect snack (carb count limit for a snack is 15 grams) and it has all the prerequisite antioxidants, vitamins and minerals to improve your health.

Adding nectarines to your regimen when they are in season means you will be better prepared to fight infections, and I can't emphasize enough about how important folic acid is for women in their reproductive years. Ladies, even if you don't plan to get pregnant, use a variety of foods – nectarines being one of them – that have high amounts of folic acid. This ensures a lower likelihood of neural tube defects – which have no cure – when you are ready to bear children.

Smooth Stalker

(Blood pressure regulator, cholesterol control, energy, immunity, anti-inflammatory, folic acid booster)

1 fresh celery rib
2 cups of butter lettuce
1 whole cucumber
1 pear (choose your favorite)

Calorie and Nutrition Count

Calories - 110
Carbs - 19g
Protein - 3g
Fiber - 5g
Vitamin A - 74mg
Vitamin C - 10mg

Ingredient Spotlight

Cantaloupe

One of the most widely available melons in the U.S., cantaloupe is off the Richter scales when it comes to potassium levels and it's even on the recommended food list for diabetics. That's a rarity for diabetics since fruits are typically high in sugar -- even though it's natural sugar -- and diabetics typically don't metabolize sugar well enough. Not so in the case of cantaloupe!

With only 16 g of carbs per serving (1 cup), cantaloupe is full of Vitamins A and C as well. Since Vitamin C acts as an antioxidant, you're aligning yourself with benefits such as anti-carcinogenic properties, as well as building up your immunity through the increase of white blood cells. Better eye health and improved skin are other reported benefits of eating the fleshy meat of the cantaloupe as well.

Another great benefit of adding cantaloupe to your diet is being able to enjoy it no matter the season. At least I've noticed this to be true as I simply love cantaloupe for breakfast and I shop for it whether there is snow on the ground or flowers in bloom.

Plum Good

(Fatigue, hangover relief, headache relief, digestion, blood sugar regulator)

½-cup red seedless grapes
½ jicama
1-cup spinach

Calorie and Nutrition Count

Calories - 186
Carbs - 40g
Protein - 5g
Fiber - 19g
Vitamin A - 57mg
Vitamin C - 123mg

Ingredient Spotlight

Grapes

In the summertime, I like to freeze my grapes whole or slice them in half, and freeze them with freshly juiced apples in ice trays with a dash of lemon juice. I will either use them, at some point, in a smoothie, a slushy drink or pop the cube in my mouth for a quick cool down and refresher after my workout session.

Grapes are a great way to combat fatigue and even migraines, not to mention being a great remedy for hangovers. Drink the juice first thing in the morning, or at the onset of a migraine without mixing it with water to get the full benefit and relief as quickly as possible.

A host of other benefits, including protection, prevention and reduction of blood clots, constipation, osteoporosis and bacterial infections result from enjoying a serving of grapes or adding them to your green smoothies.

Pear-fection

(Energy, digestion, metabolism booster, electrolyte balance, good fats, heart health)

¼-cup chopped walnuts
½-cup fresh shredded (unsweetened) coconut
8 oz. coconut Water
1 pear

Calorie and Nutrition Count

Calories 469
Carbs - 42g
Protein - 8g
Fat - 34g
Fiber - 11g
Vitamin A - 1mg
Vitamin C - 14mg

Ingredient Spotlight

Coconut sugar

With only 12 grams of carbs and a mere 45 calories per tablespoon serving, coconut palm sugar has a low glycemic index and tastes just as good, if not better than table sugar and sugar substitutes. You get the benefit of a sweetener that won't raise your blood sugar levels and it's a natural sweetener that is derived from the sap of the coconut palm tree.

With very small amounts of vitamins and minerals, coconut palm sugar can't claim to be nutrient dense, but even the trace amounts of zinc, magnesium, potassium, iron, copper phosphorus and Vitamin C put coconut palm sugar a head and shoulders beyond table sugar, which delivers no nutritional value at all.

Red Light Special

(Aphrodisiac, energy, anti-inflammatory, pH balance, lactic acid buildup relief)

2-cups watermelon
2-inch piece of ginger (about 10 slivers)
1tsp. vanilla extract
1-cup spinach
½ medium cucumber
¼-cup lemon juice
2 ounces filtered water
Splash of seltzer water (after ingredients have been blended)

Calories and Nutrition Count

Calories - 146
Carbs - 36g
Protein - 3g
Fiber - 2g
Vitamin A - 76mg
Vitamin C - 101mg

Ingredient Spotlight

Maca Powder

If you want a burst of energy, if you want to increase fertility, in both men *and* women, maca is the plant-based food you want to incorporate into your diet. Maca has been used to increase stamina as well, but maca is reported to be so potent you want to really use caution when using it.

Maca root is coming to the mainstream because, once again, anything that adds more energy to your life automatically qualifies for consideration. Add an increase in sex-drive to the mix and you've got the makings of a food that can be just about everything to everybody.

Relax! The Bloat Buster

(Digestion, blood pressure reducer, pH balance restoration, anti-inflammatory, menstrual cramp relief)

1 small honey crisp apple (or choose your favorite)
2-inch piece of ginger
½ small fennel bulb
2 ribs celery
8 ounces alkaline water (8-9.5pH)

Calorie and Nutrition Count

Calories -131
Carbs - 32g
Protein - 1g
Fiber - 8g
Vitamin A - 6mg
Vitamin C - 34mg

Ingredient Spotlight

Fennel

Whether you're bloated, constipated or just have a lot of gas that needs to get out of your system, fennel has been used for centuries as a digestive aid. Fennel is even safe enough for babies.

Women in their reproductive years will find fennel helpful as it acts to help calm some symptoms endured during the monthly cycle. Besides that, fennel is useful in so many ways, there's no reason not to add it to your diet. Of particular interest is its ability to reduce some effects of chemotherapy. For those already fighting cancer, fennel has actually been reported to reduce some of the effects of radiation treatments taken to blast away cancer cells, such as nausea, vomiting and diarrhea.

Beddie Bye

(Insomnia, heart health, anti-inflammatory, folic acid)

8 ounces unsweetened tart cherry juice
1-cup spinach
2 tbsp. sunflower seeds

Calorie and Nutrition count

Calories - 320
Carbs - 42g
Protein - 8g
Fiber - 1g
Fat - 15g
Vitamin A - 40mg
Vitamin C - 11mg

Ingredient Spotlight

Apples

They have to be my all-time favorite fruit. My favorite variety is honey crisp apples and I'm so glad to find out it's okay to have 2 apples a day. I love them with a serving of peanut butter and the health benefits I've noticed are worth the $3.99 per pound (and sometimes per apple!) price tag on them. Do I start with the fiber content (4g) or do I start with the heart disease benefits? It doesn't matter where I start. You get my drift. Apples contain Quercetin, which prevents heart disease by preventing bad cholesterol from sticking to the walls of your arteries.

Apples are also good for digestive issues, such as constipation and diarrhea. They're a low calorie treat, and relatively low-carb at 21g per medium apple, but depending on your favorite variety, apples can taste really sweet. The honey crisp apples taste like a combination of sweet and tart to me, although not everyone agrees.

Even though I do juice apples, I buy so many of them, I have enough to juice and use as the liquid base for my smoothies as well as eating them whole with a serving of peanut butter, as I mentioned above. I even freeze the juice in ice cube trays to have alone. Sometimes I add the apple cubes to other drinks for a refreshing change of pace in flavor without artificial sweeteners.

Say What! Punch

(Blood pressure/sugar regulator, immunity, weight management, eyesight protectant, breath refresher, digestion)

½ beet
½ pear (choose your favorite)
1 orange carrot
1/3 cup Goji Berries
Juice of 1 fresh lemon
½-cup fresh cilantro
2-cups spinach
10 ounces alkaline water
Add ice cubes to chill

Calorie and Nutrition Count

Calories - 155
Carbs - 36g
Protein - 5g
Fiber - 8g
Vitamin A - 317mg
Vitamin C - 64mg

Ingredient Spotlight

Wheatgrass

I promise, I didn't deliberately save the wheatgrass for last, but I think it's so appropriate since I'm a bit obsessed with it. After finding The Wheatgrass Book, by Ann Wigmore, my perception of nutrition was changed forever. I began to grow my own wheatgrass and when I needed a break, I would find it at the local health food store in liquid form as well as tablets and powders. Then I decided to create my own nutritional supplement, featuring wheatgrass as it has truly changed my health, for the better.

Wheatgrass contains chlorophyll, vitamins, minerals and live enzymes. These are all nutrients traditionally and scientifically credited as being necessary for optimal health. Chlorophyll -- specifically -- makes the blood more oxygen-rich. When the blood has more oxygen, it pumps better and carries more nutrients to all of the cells in your body. When the cells have more nutrients, they perform better and you experience higher energy level and an overall improved state of health. There may be wheatgrass naysayers, but the benefits I've personally noticed from adding wheatgrass to my diet can't be denied.

****

I've run out of room, but now that you've tried over 60 of my recipes, you've graduated to the "Green Smoothie Connoisseur" level. I hope I've helped you find your own *Green Smoothie Bliss!*

You've been exposed to new flavors in different combinations and you've formed your own opinion about what you like and what you might tweak to make it suit your particular taste buds.

There is nothing wrong with experimenting. I encourage you to switch it up a little, take these recipes I've provided for you and chop them up; maybe you'll take ½ of the ***choco-band-a-licious smoothie*** recipe and mix it with the chocolate cream supreme…who knows?

It's in your hands now. You can mix and match these recipes until your heart (and your taste buds) is content. That's part of the fun of it all. You benefit by delighting your taste buds ***and*** your heart. Be good to both…they're the only ones you have!

I hope you will join the **Live Younger, Longer and Prettier** community. The next book in the series, **Meatless Maven(s)**, will focus on even more varieties of healthier eating practices. **Meatless Maven(s)** explores more food categories like soup, ice cream, side dishes, crockpot meals, appetizers and more that are just as delicious without animal protein. No eggs, butter, milk or meat products are used to prepare the deliciousness I have in store for you in this one!

The sinfully tasty and nutritious goodies, such as my sweet potato pie smoothie, black bean burger deluxe and lasagna are all waiting for you in **Meatless Maven(s)**! All with the wellness flair that will allow you to enjoy delicious food and feel like you're treating yourself without all the guilt, calories and carbs you don't need. Can't wait to share those recipes with you!

Til we meet again,

Cheers to living younger, longer and prettier!

Coming Soon

Green Smoothie Bliss Probiotic Nutritional supplement powder

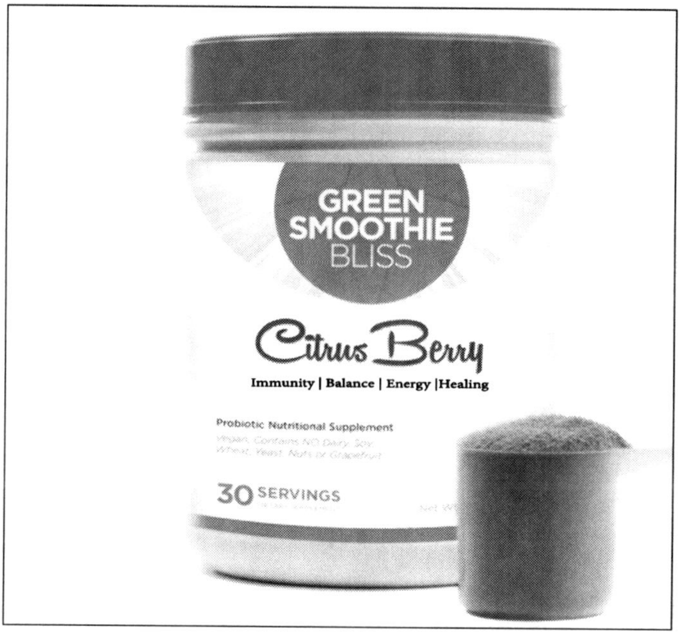

This whole food supplement has been in the developmental stages for over two years and it's finally perfect. Each flavor has a different potency level to meet you where you are on your probiotic journey. If you're just starting out, it's best to start with the lowest potency. This allows your body to properly adjust to what will be happening inside.

What will be happening, you ask? Your body will be getting assistance with digestion, building your immunity and balancing your pH -- all the things you need to promote healing, strength, immunity and balance, which will improve your health and help you get your life back. In addition, I've incorporated Amino Acids for those who struggle with low energy and lactic acid build up after working out as well as working on those awful food cravings, which can put a hell of a crimp in your plans to lose weight, if you are plagued with cravings for sweets.

Check with your doctor before consumption.

References

Institute of Medicine

University of Maryland Medical Center – Complementary & Alternative Medicine Guide

International Sports Sciences Association: Nutrition, The Complete Guide

U.S. Nutrient Database

The Wheatgrass Book by Ann Wigmore

Medline Plus

National Institute of Medicine

Natural Medicines Comprehensive Database

The Journal of Agricultural and Food Chemistry

National Institute of Health

American Chemical Society

National Center for Complementary and Alternative Medicine

The Hippocrates Institute

Scientific American

Cleveland Clinic

Whole Grains Council

Mayo Clinic

Index

CPSIA information can be obtained at www.ICGtesting.com
Printed in the USA
BVOW04s1052121114

374754BV00002B/476/P